ACT 50 THINK 40 FEEL 30

The Doctor's Secrets to Living Younger Everyday

By Allan Spreen, M.D.

with Michele Cagan

Agora Health Books
Baltimore, Maryland

Allan Spreen, M.D. with Michele Cagan
Act 50, Think 40, Feel 30...The Doctor's Secrets to Living Younger Everyday

Published by Agora Health Books

Michele Cagan, Managing editor
Ken Danz, Copy editor

ISBN 978-1-891434-28-0
Printed in the United States of America

Cover and book design by Gerrit Wessendorf

Agora Health Books
819 North Charles Street
Baltimore, Maryland 21201
www.AgoraHealthBooks.com

For additional copies of this book call 1-888-821-3609.

Act 50, Think 40, Feel 30…

The Doctor's Secrets to Living Younger Everyday

By Allan Spreen, M.D.

with Michele Cagan

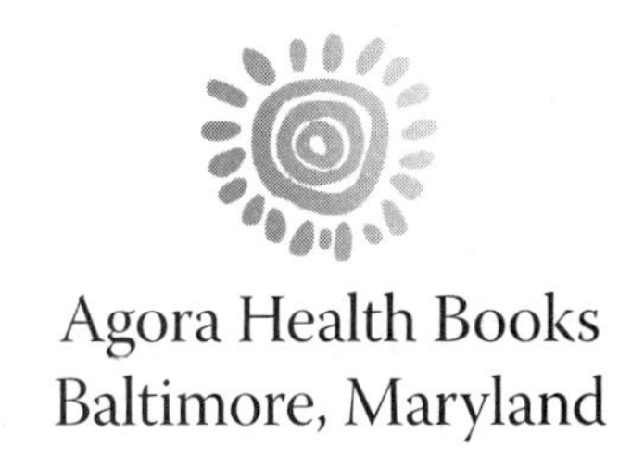

Agora Health Books
Baltimore, Maryland

DISCLAIMER

All material in this publication is provided for information only and may not be construed as medical advice or instruction. No action should be taken based solely on the contents of this publication; instead, readers should consult appropriate health professionals on any matter relating to their health and well-being.

The information and opinions provided in this book are believed to be accurate and sound, based on the best judgment available to the author, but readers who fail to consult with appropriate health authorities assume the risk of any injuries. The publisher is not responsible for errors or omissions.

THE INFORMATION PRESENTED HERE HAS NOT BEEN EVALUATED BY THE U.S. FOOD AND DRUG ADMINISTRATION. THIS PRODUCT IS NOT INTENDED TO DIAGNOSE, TREAT, CURE, OR PREVENT ANY DISEASE.

TABLE OF CONTENTS

You Have to Get Older... But You Don't Have to Age

Certain words make me cringe: *senior...elderly...decline...slowdown,* all words closely linked to aging. Just like you (and everyone else), I'm getting older. But I see myself as youthful and vital, with many enjoyable years ahead of me—no matter what my calendar says. Problem is, my body isn't always in agreement with my thoughts. I may feel 35 in my mind, but my knees and hair just don't see it that way.

You can't avoid getting older—that's purely a function of the clock. You can, however, sidestep (or at least slow down) the aging process. Sure, all of our bodies are going to age, but necessarily at the same pace or at the same point. We have a great deal of control over how quickly or slowly we age—it's almost all based on how we live.

This "new math" (calendar age vs. biological age) has been hitting the mainstream media with fists of fury—after all, there's big money to be had if you can tell people how to live longer and look younger. Make it easy, say with a single pill or injection, and you could make a fortune, even though there's no proven magic potion out there. If there were, I'd be on the beach in Bali instead of in front of a computer screen telling you the truth. It is possible to beat the clock, but you can't do it with just one little blue pill or a special hormone shot.

The secret to staying young is that there is no one big secret. Instead, there are dozens of little things you can do every day to slow down that body clock. Most of them are so easy you won't even notice the change after a couple of days. And some take a bigger commitment...but may pay out bigger results.

The first step is knowing what causes biological aging and what happens when it kicks in. Next, you need to take a look at your own body and your own health to see where preventive or reversal measures will do the most good. You'll find specific solutions for the many areas of aging—from sharpening vision to restoring full cognitive capacity to reheating-up the bedroom. You'll look younger and feel revitalized—and possibly add years to your life.

The Three Main Causes of Aging

From a biological perspective, there are three major causes of cellular aging:

- fluctuating hormone levels
- oxidative stress
- chronic inflammation

Fortunately, you can meet each of these threats head on...and stop them, or at least substantially slow them down.

Fluctuating Hormone Levels

Your body creates hormones to keep all of its organs in good working order. For many hormones, though, production levels slack off as we age. Some scientists think that decline con-

Thirty Seconds of Biology

Your body is made up of cells. Almost every cell divides to create new cells (a process called replication), and each division causes one part of the cell—called the telomere—to get smaller. When a cell's telomere shrinks to nothing, the cell can't replicate anymore; at that point, the cell dies.

Telomere is becoming a big buzzword in the world of antiaging research—you'll start hearing more about it in the mainstream any day now. Researchers have found that shorter telomeres are linked to shorter lives. So if there are two people of the same chronological age with different telomere lengths, the guy with the longer telomeres is likely to live longer. On top of that, shorter telomeres are also linked with the outward signs of aging, like gray hair.

Some scientists believe that lengthening telomeres could effectively lengthen the average human lifespan—by as much as 30 years! No one yet knows exactly how to accomplish this, or whether it will actually work.

tributes to the aging process, and that restoring hormone levels may turn back that biological clock—or at least stop it for a while.

Some of the key hormone levels that have a close link to aging include:

- testosterone
- DHEA
- human growth hormone (HGH)

Testosterone is a lot more than just a trigger for the male sex drive. For both women and men, this critical hormone supplies strength and energy (and, of course, libido). It may also help prevent diabetes, Alzheimer's disease, depression, and heart malfunctions. Unfortunately, old testosterone-replacement methods, along with misinformation that connects the hormone with prostate cancer, leave many conventional doctors believing that testosterone is unsafe—and it isn't. Quite the opposite is true, in fact: Maintaining healthy testosterone levels may prevent disease and delay aging.

DHEA is one of the lesser-known hormones, or at least it used to be. Now, it's being hyped by the antiaging crowd as a miracle youth hormone. Not quite...but when used *properly* it can help de-age several natural processes. For one thing, your body needs plentiful supplies of DHEA to make other hormones, like estrogen and testosterone. And some studies have shown that DHEA supplementation may cut down the risk of developing certain cancers.

Human growth hormone is getting even more attention than DHEA. Claims of stronger muscles, decreased body fat, and abundant energy are becoming more commonplace, and more people are injecting HGH into their bodies in an attempt to restore youth. On top of the extreme cost (treatment can run in the thousands each month), no one knows what kind of harm long-term hormone injections can do to adults.

You can maintain youthful hormone levels—but it's not as easy as just taking a pill or getting a shot and then walking away years younger. Hormone "overdose" can be more dangerous than depletion—and no one should take hormones they don't need. Plus, most doctors prescribe synthetic hormones, and those can bring on unwanted consequences. Taking the right amounts of the right hormones in the right form can help turn back the clock...but you won't find that solution in any old doctor's office.

Oxidative Stress

When metals are exposed to too much oxygen, they rust—that's oxidative damage. A similar process goes on inside our bodies. We don't actually rust from the inside out, but oxidative stress does damage our cells—aging them more quickly and contributing to disease.

The whole process starts when substances called free radicals are allowed to, well, roam free. As our bodies metabolize food, the byproducts include free radicals. At the same time, our bodies call on antioxidants—compounds from the foods we eat—to neutralize those free radicals. Antioxidants include vitamins (like A, C, and E), minerals (like selenium), and even some enzymes. Without enough antioxidant supplies, the free radicals take over and wear down our bodies one cell at a time.

But simply swallowing a handful of antioxidants every day won't turn back the clock. The trick is in knowing which ones to take and when and how to take them. Just as important is knowing which ones to take *together* and which ones to take hours apart to optimize absorption and utilization. All that information hasn't made its way into the mainstream just yet, where the focus seems to be on one or two antioxidants at a time—and usually in unnecessary megadoses.

Taken correctly, though, antioxidants appear to protect your body in innumerable ways—like warding off cataracts, boosting immunities, strengthening bones, even possibly preventing some forms of cancer. Plus, antioxidants may help your cells better repair themselves when damage does occur.

Chronic Inflammation

Most people associate inflammation with pain, and for good reason—it often comes along with injuries and chronic conditions like arthritis. But now we know that inflammation plays a much bigger role in our lives...and deaths. New research shows that inflammation plays a part in many pathological conditions, from allergies to aneurisms to Alzheimer's disease...connected to many more diseases than was previously thought.

When it's working right, inflammation actually does us a service. It helps defend our bodies against danger. Fevers, for example, kill off infectious bacteria, and swelling protects broken bones. But sometimes inflammation goes too far, damaging the body it's meant to protect. Contrary to what you'd expect, big intense bouts of inflammation aren't the ones that do the most damage. Rather it's low-grade, virtually unfelt attacks—the kind that goes unnoticed but sticks around for the long haul, causing the biggest problems. It's that chronic inflammation that has been implicated in premature aging and in many of the common ailments associated with aging.

If your first instinct upon reading that is to grab some over-the-counter (or prescription) anti-inflammatory medications—don't. Even though the conventional medical community hands out those pills like candy, that doesn't mean they're safe for long-term use. In fact, most evidence is coming in to the contrary. (Remember Vioxx?) But you can get chronic inflammation under control simply, safely, and naturally—and turn back the clock at the same time.

Rewriting the Signs of Aging

Even when we combat the controllable causes of aging, our bodies still may show some of the outward signs. Time will slow some of our systems down, and that will have an impact on how we function. And there is some plain old wear and tear that comes along with years of use: Hearing slowly declines, skin loses its resilience, and joints become less flexible. But just like we can short-circuit some of the causes of aging, we can also directly affect some of the effects. In fact, there are some very simple and safe ways to circumvent the signs of aging, and even turn back your biological clock.

With the youth-restoring solutions you'll find within this book, you may be able to:

- strengthen your immune system to feel healthier every day.
- beef up your bone density and muscle mass to feel stronger every day.
- remember everything.
- sleep all night and feel energized all day.
- restore fading vision and hearing.
- look years younger.
- enjoy a robust sex life.

Start resetting your biological clock now, before another day goes by, and watch your youth and vitality come pouring back. Live longer, stronger, and younger!

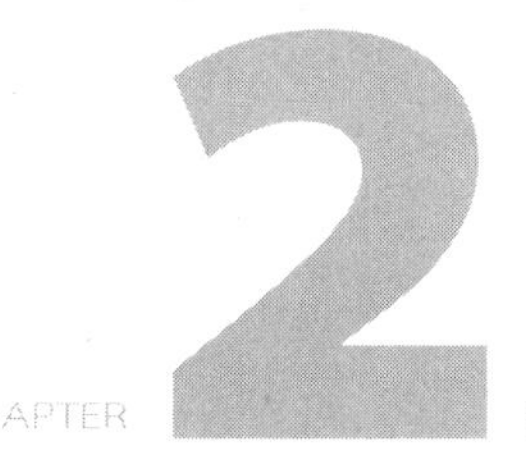

Youthful Beauty at Any Age

We all want to look younger and more beautiful—a key sign of health and vitality. But living takes a toll, and the outside may be the first place it shows up. Skin starts wrinkling and sagging, hair starts graying or (even worse) falling out. Body weight shifts, until the shape we're in doesn't remotely resemble the shape we want.

Some people turn right to surgery, for what they think are quick and easy solutions. But the most successful cosmetic surgeons are the ones with repeat customers, who come back regularly for another tuck or just one more round of liposuction. And surgery is almost never quick or easy—it can be painful, recovery can take weeks or months, complications often arise, and it puts a pretty hefty dent in your retirement account.

Luckily, there are plenty of safe and natural ways to look your best, even shave years off your appearance. They may seem to take longer than surgery, but maybe not once you factor in recovery time. Even better, these solutions will boost your overall health and appearance, rather than just one small spot.

Rejuvenate the Skin You're In

Here's the good news: you have an awful lot of control over your skin's appearance. Sure, there are some factors you can't change—like your genetics, or the suntans you got when you were 16. But you do have control over the factors that affect your skin right now:

- sun exposure
- diet
- exercise
- external care
- smoking

By readjusting these factors, you can bring back youthful skin…firmer, healthier, and (mostly) wrinkle-free. But to do that, you have to understand a few facts about your body's largest organ. (Yes, it is your skin.) First, to maintain young-looking skin on the outside, you have to build it up from the inside. Second, we now have lots of safe ways to refresh surface skin, bringing back a smooth wrinkle-free appearance. Third, we know what to avoid to prevent older-looking skin from making a comeback.

Let's tackle number three first. There's a pretty well-known list of things to avoid if you want your skin to look young and healthy:

1. too much sun
2. smoking
3. junk food

To save your skin, you have to keep these in the never-to-hardly-ever range. That doesn't mean you have to avoid sun and junk food entirely—it just means be reasonable. And on the food front, there are actually foods you can eat that can counteract the stresses of aging and keep you looking as young as you feel. As for smoking, though, quitting (as tough as that is) can only help you…no two ways about it.

Now let's talk about skin "resurfacing solutions," as I saw them called in a brochure my aunt had lying around. You've got your exfoliants, which help slough off the top layer of skin, allowing new skin to grow and show. You've got your prescription creams (tretinoin, popularly sold as Retin-A) and your over-the-counter creams (alpha-hydroxy acids, or AHAs) that also help your skin shed that damaged outer layer. And you've got procedures like chemical peels and microdermabrasion.

The first two methods (exfoliation and creams) have been used safely for years, with pretty good track records. They work well to keep your skin looking smoother and clearer, and they help fade dark spots. For fine lines and wrinkles, these products may be all you need. But when it comes to ironing out deeper wrinkles, you may need to pull out bigger guns—and that may mean a visit to a skin specialist. While you can actually buy products and try them at home, I've never seen the results of a do-it-yourself treatment turn out as well as when the same was performed by a dermatologist. (Besides, then it might be covered by your insurance company.)

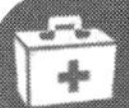

The Doctor Is In

Whether you've got a prescription from the dermatologist or a nonprescription wrinkle-minimizing cream, you must be more careful about sun exposure. Both can make your skin far more susceptible to sun damage and sunburn. If you're using one of these creams and you must spend time out in the sun, use a strong sun **block** (as opposed to sunscreen) that protects against both UVA and UVB rays and wear a wide-brimmed hat.

Let's start with chemical peels, where a chemical solution is applied directly to your face to take off the damaged top layer of skin. These have become very popular, despite the immediate "hideout" period: After the peel, your skin will probably be very red and irritated, and that can take a day or two to settle down. If you can stand that, chemical peels are a very effective way to strip off wrinkles. In most cases, you'll need a treatment about once a month.

Next up is microdermabrasion, a kinder, gentler version of traditional dermabrasion. In this process, a rotating brush with little crystals is used to polish your skin. It can reach deeper layers of skin than the other methods mentioned so far, so it can treat deeper wrinkles. The micro version uses smaller crystals, so it's not as uncomfortable or traumatic for your skin. With this method, you may be able to go three or four months between treatments.

At the far (and most expensive) end of the scale is the face-lift. This complex surgery may remove bags and sags, at least for a good long while. But it is still surgery, and comes with all the dangers inherent in any operation. My take: Talk to a plastic surgeon only after you've tried the other, much safer options.

A Word About Botox

Yes, I know Botox is FDA-approved. And I know that many people have used it to erase wrinkles, with no problem. But here's what I say about that: It's POISON, and you're getting POISON injected into your face. Even though there are plenty of "success" stories, there are plenty of potential dangers too. Earlier good luck with the procedure doesn't protect you from future problems. All it takes is a shot that misses the mark, and you've got a disfigured face (probably just temporary, but still something to consider).

The Latest Way to Smoother Skin

There used to be only two ways to deal with wrinkles: live with them or visit a plastic surgeon. Then came Botox, which gained quickly in popularity despite potentially toxic side effects. Now there's a fourth choice, one that comes with negligible side effects, minimal (if any) pain, virtually no recovery time, and smoother, younger-looking skin in no time flat. This "miracle" treatment is facial acupuncture, and I recommend it for anyone who wants to erase wrinkles.

Facial acupuncture works by balancing the Qi (life energy) in your body. Tiny needles are inserted directly into wrinkles to help restore blood flow and Qi to the spot. Each treatment takes only about 30 minutes, and it often takes more than one session for noticeable results.

Some practitioners also offer facial massage and herbal masks as part of an overall treatment, which increases the session time to about an hour. But that's a far cry from the time it takes to get, and recover from, either Botox or surgery... and there's typically no facial swelling involved. Plus, while the time-saving aspect is a definite bonus, the money-saving aspect is even better. Plastic surgery can cost thousands of dollars, and one round of Botox can set you back about $400, but facial acupuncture typically costs only $40 to $75 per treatment.

Erase Varicose Veins

Varicose veins can be troubling—especially for those of you who like to show off your legs. But you can combat this unsightly ailment with a miraculous (and very safe) herbal supplement, called gotu kola. A recent Italian study found that taking gotu kola for just two months led to noticeable improvements in vein function...and minimized the appearance of varicose veins. It works by beefing up circulation and by strengthening the tissue around the veins, keeping those veins in better shape. You can safely take up to 800 mg of the whole crude herb in capsule form, three times a day.

The Healthy Skin Diet

When it comes to feeding your face, some foods are more important than others to keep your skin looking smooth and supple. Fruits and vegetables contain antioxidants that counteract the effect of free radicals, which can cause a lot of damage to your skin. Fibrous foods can help detoxify your body, so toxins don't flow out through your pores causing damage. The "good" fats can replenish your skin and plump it up from the inside out so that wrinkles are less apparent.

Of course, when it comes to foods, some are better than others at achieving these specific goals. The very best are listed below. Here's a beautiful-skin grocery list that you can copy down and carry with you every time you go to the store:

- ❑ red grapefruit
- ❑ lemons
- ❑ berries
- ❑ dark, leafy greens (shopper's choice)
- ❑ broccoli
- ❑ whole-grain bread
- ❑ walnuts
- ❑ wild salmon

- ❑ flaxseed (or flaxseed oil)

Adding these foods to your regular diet—and cutting way back on junk—can bring about a noticeable improvement in your skin's appearance, but it will take some time (months, not days). Even better, though, it will arm your body to fight against new damage and may slow down additional signs of aging.

Supplements for Supple Skin

In some cases, foods alone can't provide enough of specific nutrients, unless you plan on eating more than your weight in produce. So on top of eating skin-healthy foods, consider taking some of these supplements to help keep your skin looking young and supple. Most of these are taken like regular vitamins, but some can work even better topically, de-aging your skin from the outside in.

There have been some very promising studies done on the topical application of antioxidants, suggesting a more dramatic impact than you'd see by taking dietary supplements. When you put antioxidants directly on your skin, they go straight to the problem and deactivate the free radicals that add to the appearance of aging—no long journey through the digestive tract first, where the antioxidants may be hijacked by other body systems that need them.

Let's work from the inside out, here, and tackle the dietary supplements first. If you aren't getting a lot of omega-3 fatty acids from food—and don't like fish or flaxseed—go for fish oil supplements. In fact, even if you do eat fish or flaxseed, you can still take a 1,000 mg capsule every day to ensure your skin gets the biggest benefit. Next, add some coenzyme Q10 (usually called coQ10). CoQ10 is a powerful antioxidant naturally produced by your body, but supplies dwindle as the years go by. Taking 60 mg of CoQ10 every day boosts your levels, helping to protect against cell damage and tighten up your skin. Now it's time to bring an essential amino acid into the mix: L-glutamine. This is another of those nutrients your body can produce itself, but production slacks off over time. Since one of L-glutamine's main jobs is keeping up collagen levels—critical for beautiful skin—a deficiency can make your skin look older. To rebuild collagen, take 500 mg of L-glutamine twice a day, away from food (meaning at least one hour before eating, or two hours after).

Now, let's head out to the surface, where some supplements work even better. Like Vitamin C: Several studies have uncovered new benefits of topical Vitamin C (usually in the form of ascorbic acid). Turns out that this powerful antioxidant, when applied to your skin, can:

- effectively minimize the appearance of facial wrinkles
- promote collagen production
- lighten up dark spots
- reduce inflammation (like from pimples)
- provide photoprotection from both UVA and UVB rays

Not all preparations are created equal, though. Vitamin C is air soluble, meaning it starts breaking down when exposed to air. On top of that, some formulations don't penetrate your skin enough to make a real difference. Ask your dermatologist about combination creams—such as Vitamin C plus retinol, proven to work together to reverse the signs of aging.

Other good topical nutrients include Vitamin E, long-used on burns and cuts to prevent scarring. Now we know that it can also reduce fine lines on your face as well. This antioxidant appears to work best when the preparation is based on the alpha-tocopherol form of Vitamin E, so look for that on the label. For sagging skin, try applying a DMAE preparation—it won't erase wrinkles, but it may firm up your cheeks and jowls. Be prepared for some sticker shock, though: Compared with the other creams mentioned here, those containing DMAE may seem pretty pricey.

Hair Where You Want It (And Not Where You Don't)

Changes in your hair are among the more noticeable signs of aging—thinning, breaking off, falling out. Most people believe those changes are inevitable and uncontrollable, but they're wrong. Sure, you can't change your age or your genetics, but you can take some very simple steps to help minimize, or even reverse, some of those problems.

Your hair is directly affected by your overall health. A change in your well-being can bring on changes in your hair—things like extra stress, or nutritional deficiencies (often caused by dieting), or an unreliable thyroid. Plus, lots of people have external hair-destroyers to deal with, like chemotherapy.

There are a couple of over-the-counter drugs out there to restore hair loss: minoxidil and finasteride (the second is approved only for use by men). Both drugs promote hair growth due to normal male pattern baldness; minoxidil can also be used for extreme hair thinning experienced by women. Once you start taking these drugs, you're stuck with them...the minute you stop taking the pills, your newly grown hair will disappear.

If taking hair-growth drugs or going the fake-hair route doesn't appeal to you, you can try some natural solutions. Specific supplements work to improve your overall health, and better hair is a wonderful side effect of that. These particular supplements send much-needed nutrients to your hair through the roots, helping you build up a healthier head of hair. And if you have been using minoxidil or finasteride, these supplements can work right along with them.

- Zinc can produce healthy hair and may even slow down hair loss. This mineral works especially well for people experiencing underactive thyroid, which can lead to brittle or thinning hair. Take 30 mg of zinc every day, and you may notice a difference in just a few weeks. **A word from the doctor:** Whenever you increase your zinc, add in some copper to balance it out. For a 30-mg dose of zinc, add 2 mg of copper to your daily regimen.

- Biotin, part of the B-vitamin family, is a known hair restorer. Not only can this essential nutrient stall hair loss and strengthen your hair, but it may also actually bring on new hair growth—when the loss was caused by a biotin deficiency, that is. Biotin works best when it's joined by the rest of the B-vitamin clan, so look for it in a B complex that contains 50 mcg of biotin.

- PABA (a.k.a. para-aminobenzoic acid), another member of the

> B-vitamin lineup, also plays a role in hair protection. PABA protects your hair through its roots, and getting enough of this critical nutrient can keep your hair from falling out. Make sure your B complex contains 100 mg of PABA.

As for herbs, there are a couple that have been shown to help. Saw palmetto, sometimes used to treat an enlarged prostate, may also fight male pattern baldness, thanks to its ability to dampen down the effects of testosterone. Pygeum africanum also appears to do the trick for male pattern baldness, probably by that same mechanism. You can add 160 mg of saw palmetto and 100 mg of pygeum to your daily regimen to fight hair loss. Oh, and ladies, these just may work for you as well.

For the other side of the hormone coin, there are some Chinese herbs that can prevent hair loss by boosting the power of estrogen. Those traditional herbs include dong quai and shou wu. You can take 500 mg three times a day of both these herbs. You can take them together; in fact, you may be able to find one product that contains both herbs.

The Iron Connection

Some innovative new research uncovered a very surprising fact: Iron deficiency plays a big role in hair loss. And taking in more iron could play a big role in regrowth. Especially for women, supplementing with iron can stall hair shedding and maximize growth potential.

You don't have to have full-blown anemia for your hair to be affected, either. In fact, that's one of the biggest misconceptions the researchers came across. The iron deficiencies that can leave more hair in the sink then on your head are much smaller than the ones that lead to anemia.

But here's a word of warning: Don't stock up on the iron supplements until you see a doctor and get a blood test. Taking too much iron when your body already has plenty can lead to iron overload...a pretty dangerous condition. Besides, a lot of people have a hard time tolerating iron supplements, as they can cause stomach upset and constipation. You may have better luck just adding iron-rich foods to your diet, without any of the uncomfortable side effects and potential dangers. Good food sources include:

- lentils
- oysters
- prunes
- raisins
- spinach
- beef (lean cuts are best)

To absorb the most iron from your meals, eat foods rich in Vitamin C along with the foods listed above. Vitamin C helps your body absorb iron more easily.

Hairy Hormones

Hormone levels dip as we get older, and among the most noticeable are estrogen and testosterone levels. Those hormones are what separate the men from the girls, in more ways than one. Like this: Testosterone is responsible for more, thicker hair all over. Estrogen holds off testosterone, giving women finer body hair. With time, women's estrogen levels drop just like men's testosterone levels. In men, that shows up as a little less body hair and a lot less hair on the head. Women may experience thinner and thinning hair on their heads. . . and the addition of (unwanted) manlike hair in other places, like the upper lip or chest. Returning hormone levels to earlier norms can prevent or reverse these effects in many cases—but don't overdo it, or you'll be buying more problems than you've bargained for.

Say Goodbye to Gray

When your hair fades to gray, you can decide to live with it or start coloring it. Or you can try some basic supplements that may just restore vibrant hair color on their own. When you're looking to restore color, your best bet is to do it gradually so that it looks like a natural process. That's the effect you'll see if supplements can do the trick, and the effect you want if color-in-a-box is the ticket.

Copper plays a crucial role in hair color—no matter what color that is. Your body needs copper in order to produce a compound called melanin, the pigment responsible for your skin and hair color. Without enough copper, you can't produce enough melanin, and your hair could begin to lose its color. This condition is extremely common in people who take zinc supplements, because zinc blocks copper absorption. When copper deficiency is the culprit, supplements can turn things around and bring back your natural hair color. All it takes is 2 mg a day (best taken at least two hours before or after any zinc supplements).

PABA is another nutrient involved in your hair color. When you don't get enough of this B vitamin, your hair may turn gray. But adding it to your supplement regimen may reverse the graying process. Take 100 mg of PABA daily—even better, take it as part of an overall B complex supplement.

In China, Siberian ginseng has been used for generations to prevent the gray hair that comes with age. Possibly due to some estrogen-like qualities, this traditional herb may just do the trick if your fading hair color has a hormone-based cause. You can safely take up to 600 mg per day. To maximize this powerful herb's effectiveness, take a two-week break (where you stop taking Siberian ginseng) every three months. **A note from the Doctor:** Make sure you get Siberian ginseng, not Panax or American.

The Dirt on Dyes

Using hair color is a great option if you want to get rid of the gray—we've been doing it for centuries, with great results. It was only during the past century that permanent dyes came into being, and those are the ones that may pose some dangers. Several permanent dyes contain known or suspected carcinogenic ingredients...and the worst appear to be in dark hair colors. That doesn't mean you can't or shouldn't color your hair. It just means that you should consider safer alternatives like natural, temporary, or semipermanent dyes. (Yes, you'll have to color more often, but the trade-off is cancer protection.)

Tone, Tighten, and Take Off Pounds

Accept it: You can't look or feel your best unless you exercise. Keeping your body in tiptop shape requires some form of physical activity, done on a regular basis. Now, I know it can be hard to drag yourself away from the screen—TV, computer, doesn't much matter which—but you have to get yourself moving. The results will be more than worth the effort.

If you've been sedentary for a while now, ease yourself back into an exercise routine. Start with something basic, like walking or swimming, for short periods of time (say 15 or 20 minutes to start). Before you know it, you'll be moving faster and exercising longer. You'll feel healthier and stronger all around—and your body will start to look like it did years ago.

For the best results, your workout plan needs two components: aerobic exercise and strength training. Mixing these together will give you the best body you can have: stronger, leaner, healthier. And as a bonus, many studies show that being in better shape brings on a better love life (and isn't that why we all want to look and feel better anyway?).

Aerobic Exercise

Aerobic exercise is the kind that gets your heart pumping, bringing increased oxygen into your system. To lose weight, you have to include some form of aerobic exercise in your schedule. It can be walking, swimming, dancing—whatever you like, as long as it elevates your heart rate. Just 30 minutes a day will do the trick, getting you closer to the body you had 30 years ago.

Besides giving you a beautiful body, regular aerobic exercise will show up in your face as well. Boosted circulation and plenty of oxygen go a long way toward bringing youth back to your face—some color in your cheeks, better skin tone (meaning firmness), and more vibrancy.

What counts as aerobic exercise (besides the walking, swimming, and dancing mentioned above, that is)?

- bicycling
- jogging
- water aerobics
- climbing stairs

- rowing a boat
- mowing your lawn (and yes, only using a push mower counts)
- playing tennis

Strength Training

Everyone's muscles diminish with age—everyone's. The only way to maintain muscles is to work them, but it's not as hard as you think. Strength training includes working out with weights, resistance exercise, and weight-bearing movements, and you can do whichever one you want to get great results. When you add strength training to your program, you'll get rid of body fat, add lean muscle mass, and walk taller. And all it takes is about 20 minutes, three times a week. Within the first few weeks, you'll start to feel stronger and gain stamina. And within just six months of regular strength training, you can increase your strength by 50%...making it much easier to carry in the groceries.

So, how do you get started? The latest research shows that all you need to do is one set of 12 repetitions at the right weight for your workout to work. You can tell you're using the right weight when you can just barely complete your last repetition. While you're searching for just the right weight, it's better to start too light than too heavy. If you have no idea where to start, go for 1-pound or 2-pound weights and work your way up from there. Oh, and remember to warm up your muscles with five minutes of brisk walking followed by a couple of minutes of stretching *before* you get started.

Better, Not Bigger

When I recommend strength training to women, they usually roll their eyes and tell me they don't want big muscles. My response: That's not going to happen, but lots of other things will. You'll get stronger and leaner. You'll burn up more calories all the time, even when you're just sitting around. And you'll protect yourself against osteoporosis, even if it has already started. You'll look and feel better, not bigger.

You can also try resistance bands, long "ropes" of stretchy plastic. These bands are very inexpensive and are available in a wide range of different tensions to match your current abilities. To work your arms, you can stand on the middle of the band and do arm curls with the ends. To work your legs, you can wrap a band around them, and then step side to side within that circle. Or for the free version of strength training, use your own body for the weight. Do push-ups or pull-ups for your arms, crunches for your abdomen, and squats for your hips and thighs.

Posture Perfect

One of the most enduring stereotypes linked to aging is the picture of a hunched-over person. You can sidestep that image with a combination of core-muscle and weight-bearing exercises. Strengthening your core muscles (abdomen, stomach, and lower-back) lends support to your spine, helping it stand straight and tall. Weight-bearing exercise strengthens your bones as well as your muscles—and you need strong bones to stand tall.

CHAPTER 3

Rev Up Your Sex Life

It doesn't matter how old you are, sex can make you feel like a kid again—and great sex can make you feel even better. As we start to age, some of our drives diminish a little bit at a time, and sex drive is one of those. Some folks may just throw up their hands and settle for less, but the rest of us look for ways to get back in the saddle again.

The first step toward the second round of a great sex life is knowing what you're up against. Some medical conditions can put a damper on desire, and medications can be even worse. In fact, the list of drugs that can potentially cause impotence is so long it could take up its own chapter. And for many people, sexual troubles start in the mind and then affect the body. Once you've figured out what's causing your difficulties, you can start dealing with the problem, and take your sex life off hold.

Let's Talk Medications

As I mentioned in the beginning of the chapter, there are dozens of medications that can interfere with your sex drive. Here's the most important thing to remember: Even if you believe one of these drugs is causing your sexual difficulties, don't

The Next Generation of ED Drugs

Viagra, Cialis...those are yesterday's news. Tomorrow's treatments offer faster, longer-lasting erections, even an almost-cure for the problem. They're nowhere near the shelves yet. They don't even have brand names yet...but you can expect to start hearing about them pretty soon.

The faster-acting pill (avanafil) doesn't last very long. That sounds like a disadvantage, but it's really a benefit for guys who can't take traditional ED drugs because they're already taking heart medications. Human trials have shown that taking avanafil in combination with nitrate-based drugs doesn't cause the sharp ups and downs in blood-pressure numbers that come with today's ED meds.

The longer-lasting erection pill (SLx-2101) gives you two drugs in one dose. The first works just like Viagra, kicking in quickly to block the enzyme that forces smooth muscles to contract. As that drug does its magic, it also produces a second dose to help keep you going longer.

The virtual "cure" (hMaxi-K) is a type of gene therapy. It enters cells and tells them to make a specific protein that tells smooth muscles it's time to relax. That lets blood flow freely into your penis, erasing a major cause of ED. This drug isn't quick-acting, or long-lasting. You don't plan to have sex, then take it. Even better—it lets your body get an erection whenever you're aroused, just like before.

These medications are still in the testing stages, so it may be a while before they're widely available. And since the testing is still in its early stages, we have almost no information about potential side effects and consequences or about interactions with other medications.

stop taking it without talking to your doctor first. Tell him what's going on, and ask if there's something else you can try that won't stick you with this very undesirable side effect.

Keep in mind that this list is not all-inclusive. Every day we're discovering new drugs, with new side effects. These are just some of the most commonly taken medications that have sexual problems among their common side effects. If you've started taking a medication that is not on this list and suddenly lose your desire or ability to enjoy sex, tell your doctor and come up with a different treatment plan.

- **antihypertensive drugs,** such as Lopressor, Dibenzaline, Serpasil, Diuril, and Lonitem

- **muscle relaxers,** such as Flexeril and Norflex
- **antianxiety drugs,** such as Librium, Valium, Tybatran
- **Tagamet**
- **Flagyl**
- **Dilantin**

Pump Up the Volume

Desire may start in your mind, but it needs cooperation from body parts to be quenched. The physical side of desire is arousal, and for that you need plenty of blood flowing. One of the key causes of flagging physical response is a plain old circulation problem—and that comes with a simple fix. Get the blood moving again, and you can get your mojo back.

It's completely physiological. No man's getting an erection without ample blood flow...no woman can experience normal arousal responses (lubrication, heightened sensitivity) when the blood flow's just not getting to the vagina. To get your mojo back, you have to pump up the volume, and get the blood flow down to where you really need it. There are lots of mainstream ways to make this happen—but I recommend the much safer and equally effective natural methods.

Niacin, a.k.a. Vitamin B3

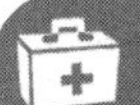

The Doctor Is In

Don't take niacin without first talking to your doctor if you have any of the following conditions: diabetes, low blood pressure, liver disease, gout, ulcers, glaucoma, or bleeding problems.

If you're looking for ways to improve your sex life, look no further than niacin. You need this essential vitamin in order to produce energy—and it takes energy to make love. Even more important, niacin acts as a vasodilator, meaning it helps keep your blood vessels wide open for maximum blood flow. That circulation boost brings plenty of flow to your nether regions, where it's needed for a satisfying sex life. Best, it works fast, in about fifteen minutes (you'll feel the tingle down below).

It can be tempting to take whopping doses of B3, but don't do it unless you want to experience some undesirable and potentially dangerous side effects. Also, stay away from time-release niacin capsules, as they've been found to cause liver damage in some cases. To get your blood flowing, all you really need is 100 mg of niacin, best taken as part of a B-complex supplement.

Vitamin E

While niacin offers an immediate response, Vitamin E is more of a long-term solution. It boosts circulation by strengthening your arteries and widening their passageways. On top of that, this nutrient strengthens your heart and boosts your stamina—it does that by squeezing every ounce of available energy out of the oxygen you take in. To get your blood moving, take 600 IU of Vitamin E twice a day.

The DHEA Link

DHEA (dehydroepiandrosterone) is the hormone we make the most of, which is true for both men and women. It's used to make a bunch of other critical hormones: corticosterone, estrogen,

The Pressure's On, Ladies

We've known for a long time that high blood pressure can cause bedroom problems for men. And now we know that women are in the same club, thanks to some new scientific research.

A recent study found that women with high blood pressure are twice as likely to be hit with sexual dysfunction than those with normal pressure readings. In fact, the researchers found that 42% of women with high blood pressure experienced sexual dysfunction. Doctors aren't exactly sure how high blood pressure affects a woman's sex drive and enjoyment...just that it can impair both.

Sounds like just controlling your blood pressure can bring back an enjoyable sex life, but the most common ways of doing that can actually cause sexual problems. Many of the drugs used to treat high blood pressure can zap your libido. So what's a woman to do? Treat her high blood pressure naturally and solve two problems at once.

Ginseng and ginger—both staples of traditional Chinese medicine—have been shown to effectively reduce high blood pressure. Another of my favorites is lemon balm. It has properties that help slightly dilate blood vessels, which, in turn, helps lower blood pressure. Lemon balm makes a tasty tea, and you can have as many as three cups a day safely.

testosterone, and progesterone. Like a lot of other things, DHEA levels drop off as we age...and by the time we hit about 65 years old, DHEA production can plummet by more than 80%. That nosedive in DHEA can cause the production of other hormones to plunge as well.

You can replenish some of that lost DHEA by taking supplements. Several human studies have been conducted, but with very different results: Some showed improved sexual function, while others showed no change. The trick is to take the right amount, and no more than that—no one has ever tested long-term use of large dosages, and I'd advise against super-high adrenal hormone levels. Try taking 25 mg per day during the week and give your body a break over the weekend to let your adrenal glands rest.

Back in Balance: Women and Hormones

It's a fact of life, ladies. Hormone levels decrease as you age, and that can cause a serious decline in your sex drive. And even when your desire remains on high, the shifting hormones can set off other problems that make sex less pleasant (sometimes actually unpleasant). Those side issues include reduced responsiveness, vaginal dryness, physical discomfort during sex, and inability to achieve orgasm.

But here's the big problem: Most hormone-replacement therapies (HRTs) out there are dangerous. Sure, they may work to ease some symptoms, but they can also cause major health problems (including cancer and heart attacks). The trick is to replace or regenerate the right hormones in the right way to get the results you want without the deadly side effects of traditional HRT. And the best way to do that is with bio-identical hormones.

You won't find bio-identical hormones every-

Sex Makes You Smarter

German researchers did their homework, and here's what they found: It seems that having sex on a regular basis can make you smarter. That's because your body produces copious quantities of adrenalin and hydrocortisone during sex...and those chemicals stimulate your brain. More brain stimulation equals a more intellectual you—so put down that crossword puzzle and get down to business.

where you look, but you can find them at special compounding pharmacies. My favorite pharmacy for true natural hormones is the Women's International Pharmacy. The pharmacists there compound the hormones you need in the form you need them—oral, topical, suppository, or sublingual—depending on your unique situation. For more information about this pharmacy, you can look at its Web site at www.womensinternational.com.

The Trouble With Testosterone

When women are having hormone problems, doctors usually jump right to estrogen. But when it comes to a lack of interest in sex, the real answer might be testosterone. See, most women find their testosterone levels dropping by anywhere from 10% to 50% by the time they hit their mid-40s, causing all sorts of undesirable consequences, like:

- less sexual desire
- reduced ability to achieve orgasm
- decreased nipple and clitoral sensitivity
- thinned pubic hair
- decreased muscle tone
- dry skin
- generally lower energy levels

Getting testosterone levels back in line can reverse some (maybe even all) of those symptoms, and rekindle sexual enjoyment.

The trick is in getting yourself to the right level and not just adding more testosterone into your system. The first step is to test your current testosterone levels. If they are below normal, you and your doctor can work to correct

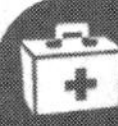

The Doctor Is In

Even if you're not experiencing any sexual problems, you could still have low testosterone levels. If you do—even if you aren't feeling any consequences—talk to your doctor about correcting them. Osteoporosis can be more of a problem when testosterone is running low, and that's a problem you definitely want to avoid.

Aphrodisiacs Anyone?

These aphrodisiacs are the foods of love, foods believed to heighten sexual arousal and enjoyment. Do they work? Some say yes, others no. I say anything that might help get you in the mood is worth trying, especially when it's part of a romantic dinner. Next time you're setting the stage for seduction, make sure some of these foods are on the menu:

- peaches
- asparagus
- caviar
- oysters
- figs
- artichokes
- avocados
- pine nuts
- mussels
- chocolate
- arugula
- basil

them. But if they do fall in the normal range, additional testosterone is not called for—even if you are having symptoms like the ones listed above. Then, the answer lies somewhere else.

The Desire Detective

Once you've ruled out hormone levels as the problem, you can turn your attention to other possible causes for your diminished desire. Believe it or not, I've found that a lot of women experience this effect from a very simple, very common problem: candidiasis (a.k.a. yeast). Candidiasis is a 'non-diagnosis' in conventional medicine (meaning they almost never consider it unless there's an obvious vaginal yeast infection). So word of mouth sent a lot of women my way, many with low sex drive near the top of the symptom list (usually falling right after fatigue). Lots of these women had been treated as if they were crazy by conventional doctors—who accused them of exaggerating, or even making up symptoms—just because those doctors couldn't figure out what was wrong. When I treated these women AS IF they had this "nonexistent" illness, at least 80% of them got much better...fatigue, flagging sex drive, headaches, and other seemingly unrelated symptoms disappeared.

Guys: Viagra's NOT the Answer

When Viagra first hit the scene, men all over hailed it as the perfect answer to the "Where'd my hard-on go?" question. They just popped a pill, waited a few minutes, and the answer was blatantly obvious. Instant arousal seemed miraculous... until the women started complaining: "He's ready to go, and I haven't even got started yet!"

And that complaint is just one drawback to the quick erection. Now consider some of the reported side effects of Viagra:

- headaches (including migraines)
- dizziness
- urinary tract infection
- diarrhea
- indigestion
- edema (swelling of the arms and legs)
- pain
- rashes
- abnormal vision changes
- heart problems (from angina to heart failure)

Sowing Your Wild Oats

Here's a little-known fact: The phrase "sowing your wild oats" has roots in sexual history. For centuries, Europeans have used wild oats for their aphrodisiac properties...for men and stallions. Fast forward to 1985, when wild oats (a.k.a. Avena sativa) were clinically tested in people. The subjects were given 300 mg of the herb for four weeks, and the results were exciting. Women reported a 21% increase in sexual thoughts and fantasies, a 19% increase in sexual satisfaction, and a 30% increase in the frequency of their sexual activity. As for the men, they reported a 25% increase in sexual pleasure and a 22% increase in genital sensitivity.

The list goes on and on, but these are some of the more commonly reported issues. Some of these are real mood killers, but that's too bad—you may not be in the mood, but your penis isn't calming down any time soon. And the last side effect is more than a mood killer; it can actually kill you.

The thing is, you don't need to suffer (or die) to have great sex again. You don't have to trade an erection for a migraine or indigestion. There are lots of natural ways to improve your sex drive, performance, and enjoyment—to enjoy easier and longer-lasting erections and more intense orgasms—without putting yourself in any danger. I'm going to tell you about the best ones, and get you back in the saddle.

Muira puama doesn't exactly roll off the tongue, but its common name says it all: potency wood. Supplements made from this Brazilian shrub increase sexual desire and erection...but they do take some time to work. One study found that

60% of patients battling impotence were able to achieve an erection within two weeks of adding the herb to their regimen. And another study found that 63% of men taking muira puama enjoyed more frequent sex. You can either take between 1 and 1.5 grams of the extract daily or drink one cup of muira puama tea each morning...but don't do both! You'll find muira puama preparations at most health-food stores.

Horny goat weed is another herb with a great name and the ability to give back your lost erections. This herb (also called barrenwort) has been used in traditional Chinese medicine for centuries as a remedy for impotence, as a premature-ejaculation preventive, and as an aphrodisiac. Horny goat weed affects your body in two key ways to achieve that sexual trifecta: It dilates blood vessels (to boost circulation) and increases levels of dopamine (a feel-good brain chemical that plays a role in testosterone release). Take 1,000 to 3,000 mg per day of horny goat weed. You should be able to find it in capsule, tablet, or powder form in most health-food stores. One note of caution: This herb is for short-term use only, so don't plan on using it for the long haul.

L-arginine is an amino acid that can give you back your erections. One of the greatest things about l-arginine is that it works with the natural processes of your body to get your sexual mojo going again. Plus, it's proven to be as effective as lots of prescription drugs without subjecting you to a laundry list of nasty side effects. There are dozens of studies showing the effects of this amino acid on male potency, making it perhaps the best thing you can take to restore your sex life—in fact, your body can not achieve erection without it! Take 1,000 to 2,000 mg every day, away from food, and you should feel it working in about two weeks.

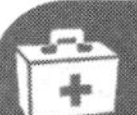

The Doctor Is In

So you don't think I'm singling out Viagra, it's fiercest competitors come with ridiculously long lists of bad side effects as well. Both Cialis and Levitra come with a lot of the same potential consequences as Viagra, and some of their own as well. Cialis has been directly linked to hypertension, heart attack, back and muscle pain, and abnormal liver function. Levitra may come with a side of nausea, heartburn , visual disturbances (blue auras, blurriness), and irregular heart beat.

Yohimbe comes with a caution: Though this

herb can do wonderful things for your sexual function, it comes with an impressive array of possible adverse side effects and health warnings, just like prescription ED drugs. For that reason, I'm extremely careful about recommending it. No one should take this herb without guidance from a medical professional. You can get the prescription version (yohimbine hydrochloride) at most pharmacies. Or you can try the nonprescription variety, the extract form. If you decide to go the non-prescription route, it's still a good idea to talk to a doctor or naturopath first. The standard dosage is 15 to 20 mg per day, but you can take up to 42 mg per day; always start with the lowest dosage and give that a chance to work. Here's one more caution: Many of the yohimbe preparations you'll find in health-food stores don't list the dosage, so get the right dosage for that formula from a naturopath or pharmacist.

Exercises for Better Sex

Exercise leads to better sex—that's the general rule, and it's really true. Exercise gets your blood flowing, and arousal is all about blood flow. Being physically fit overall will do wonders for your romantic life...and some special exercises that work out your sexual muscles can take your love life up a notch.

One big study, conducted at the Harvard School of Public Health, found that physically active men reported better erections. All it takes to make ED a thing of the past is a 30-minute walk almost every day. ED affects more than 150 million men around the world, and the No. 1 cause is vascular, accounting for about 40% of all cases. Once you get blood flowing throughout your whole body, it will make its way to your penis as well.

Ladies, this whole-body-exercise idea works just as well for you. Overall fitness, especially cardiovascular fitness, can increase your sexual desire and pleasure.

Guys: Develop Your Sexual Energy

Once your body is in great shape, it's time to focus on your pleasure centers. The more you exercise your sexual muscles (either with a partner or on your own), the better sex you'll have. Three key exercises, drawn from ancient Chinese practices, can help you develop your sexual energy...and increase sensitivity (the physical kind, not the emotional kind). These are:

- Belly Breathing
- Stopping the Stream
- PC Pull-ups

Each of these exercises can boost your sexual prowess, and when you put them together—watch out!

Keep It Big

To keep your sex life from shriveling, don't let your body shrivel! Full-body exercise is critical to keep up your sexual desire and let you enjoy rip-roaring orgasms. The best exercises are the ones that get your heart pumping: fast walking, swimming, cycling, and cross-country skiing are all great choices. Maintain your overall physical fitness (without overdoing it) and a very satisfying sex life will follow.

Belly Breathing

Strange as it sounds, strengthening your breathing is the first step toward controlling ejaculation and experiencing deeper sexual sensations. Most of us are shallow breathers, taking breaths into our shoulders and chests—but this method allows only a small amount of oxygen to be absorbed by our lungs. Belly breathing, where you breathe deeply into the bottom of your lungs and into your diaphragm, bumps up the oxygen and pumps up the stimulation.

To learn how to belly breathe, start by lying on your back with your knees bent and your feet flat on the floor (or bed). As you take a breath, focus on breathing deeply into your belly, allowing it to expand outward as you take in air. When you breathe out, let your belly deflate. Continue these belly breaths for five minutes...and expect to feel relaxed and energized when you get up.

Stopping the Stream

Next up: developing your sexual strength. To do that, you need to work your PC (pubococcygeus) muscle, which stretches from the front of your pubic bone all the way to the tailbone at the back tip of your butt. This very important muscle is the one you use to hold it in when you have to pee at an inconvenient time, and it's also the one that delivers orgasms—very important muscle.

The easiest way to work the PC muscle is to stop your urine flow right in the middle. Try to stop and start urinating as many times as you can—aim for at least three times per bathroom break. And pay attention to how you accomplish that, because it will help you work this muscle even when you don't have to pee (see below).

PC Pull-ups

To make your PC muscle even stronger—and your orgasms even better—you can use what you learned from stopping the stream even when you're not (stopping the stream, that is). Now you can contract the PC pretty much any time, anywhere...in the car, at your desk, in front of the TV. The important thing is to practice contracting and releasing that muscle as often as you can.

When PC pull-ups start to seem easy, it's time to increase the hold time of that contraction phase and the number of reps. Aim for 10 reps at a time, with each contraction held for at least a count of five. Do your pull-ups at least twice a day.

Ladies: Pleasure Starts Here

The No. 1 exercise for heightening your sexual pleasure is the Kegel. Kegel exercises are designed to strengthen the muscles that make up the pelvic floor. These exercises were originally created to help control minor urinary incontinence, very common during and after menopause. Lo and behold! A very enjoyable side effect was quickly discovered...these exercises can increase your sexual pleasure immensely.

Kegel exercises are very easy to do. To get the feel of the right muscles, stop the flow of urine midstream the next time you go to the bathroom. And pay close attention—the muscles you use to stop the stream will be the ones you'll work while doing the Kegel exercises. The trick is to target them so you can start doing the exercises wherever you are, and not just while you pee.

Every day, tighten those muscles and hold them like that for a count of four (a slow four). Then relax for a count of 10. Repeat the tighten-and-relax process 10 times, five times a day. And since no one will be able to tell that you're doing your Kegels, you can do them whenever and wherever it's convenient for you—at the checkout counter, while polishing your nails, while playing bridge. Most women report a monumental pleasure boost after about three months of daily Kegels.

Take Control of Urinary Incontinence

Even patients who've known me for decades keep quiet about overactive-bladder (OAB) or urinary-incontinence (UI) problems, so I'm always the one who brings it up. I ask questions, they look at the wall behind my head and mumble vague answers. That is, until I can convince them that those conditions are totally treatable, completely medical issues. Working together, we can make it go away.

You'd be surprised how many people suffer from incontinence every day and most of them don't realize that they're not alone. UI and OAB affect more than 13 million Americans every day, making them some of the most common conditions around. But because of the sensitive nature of the symptoms, most OAB and UI sufferers don't tell their doctors what's wrong, and they continue to go untreated.

The Top 5 Reasons People Keep Quiet About Incontinence

1. It's embarrassing.
2. It's not really a medical condition.
3. It's really a minor problem, especially compared to friends who have cancer or heart problems.

4. It's a regular, inevitable part of getting older.
5. There's nothing you can do about it anyway.

The truth is that OAB and UI are more than just physical conditions. They take a big toll on your emotional well-being too. Just think about it: How many times has fear of an incident kept you from doing something you really wanted to do or from going somewhere you wanted to go? Like taking your grandson to his first major league game, but worrying that he'll miss an astounding double play because you had to run to the bathroom and he had to come with you. Or going to the movies with your book club, and fretting that you won't be able to get the seat at the end of the aisle when you know you'll be up and down a bunch of times. A recent study found that 75% of people with OAB said that their condition got in the way of daily activities. And even with that level of discomfort and disruption, less than half of them would even think about discussing it with their doctors.

Consider this, though: In more than 80% of all cases, treatment is extremely effective. Even better, the best treatments are the ones you control—like special exercises and behavioral or dietary changes.

What You Didn't Know About Your Bladder

Your bladder has two primary jobs: storing urine at the lowest possible pressure level and getting rid of that liquid when it hits the maximum storage. Since your body produces urine *all the time* (thanks to your kidneys), those are two very important tasks. Glitches in either one of those functions can keep you running to the bathroom.

Let's Talk Biology

Though UI and OAB may seem pretty similar, the conditions are about as much alike as gorillas and grapefruits. In the case of OAB, your bladder muscles go on the blink, sending down the urgency signal even when there's really nothing much to shout about. With UI, any one of several reasons can cause urine to leak out no matter how hard you try to prevent it. Sometimes the two overlap, when an overactive bladder goes even further off the track and causes urge incontinence.

When it comes to incontinence, knowing the cause is the first step toward finding a cure. There are five basic types of UI, and each has a different source and demands a different treatment approach.

- Stress incontinence, which causes urine loss with physical exertion (anything from a single sneeze to some heavy lifting).
- Urge incontinence, which occurs when your bladder feels like it has to go right now
- Mixed incontinence, which combines the stress and urge varieties, attacking both on its own urgency schedule and with exertion
- Functional incontinence, which happens when all your plumbing is working properly but something interferes with your getting to the bathroom fast enough. This is a common prescription-drug side effect.
- Transient incontinence, which comes about when something (like illness or medication) makes your kidneys produce so much urine that the rest of your body can't keep up.

There are some causes that bridge the gender gap, but others that are strictly sex-specific. Some of the more general causes, the ones that can strike anyone, include age-related decrease in bladder capacity and function, chronic interstitial cystitis (near constant urinary infections), bladder cancer, neurological disorders (like MS and Parkinson's disease), and obstructions (like tumors and stones). In addition to victims of these direct causes, both men and women who are disabled by illness or injury also struggle with incontinence, mainly because they simply can't reach the bathroom in time.

For obstructions and infections, a visit to a urologist is called for. Medical intervention can deal with the immediate problem. Then you can work with your doctor to determine the best ways to prevent recurrences.

For Men Only

For us men, prostate problems can cause all sorts of trouble in the urination department. That's mainly because of biological geography: Your prostate sits right under your bladder and surrounds your urethra, the tube urine flows through as it travels down from the bladder and out the penis. Anytime your prostate gets enlarged, it interferes with that process and causes urinary problems.

There are three conditions that can cause an enlarged prostate. The first, prostatitis, is pretty rare, but it can affect you if you've let urinary-tract infections (like cystitis) go untreated. The condition is usually the result of a bacterial infection and can be treated with antibiotics. The second, benign prostate hyperplasia (BPH), is extremely common, especially in older men. That's because as soon as you hit 40, your prostate starts to grow, just a little—but it can be enough to squeeze your urethra and block your normal flow. The third, and most serious, is prostate cancer. Here, though, incontinence is more likely to be caused by treatment than by the disease itself.

For Women Only

One of the more common causes of incontinence in women is the big hormonal change that comes with menopause. As estrogen levels drop, the linings of your bladder and urethra lose some of their natural elasticity. That makes it harder for those tissues to close when they're supposed to, so they can't hold back urine as easily as they did before.

A hysterectomy can also trigger urinary incontinence. Again, this is a function of biological geography. Your uterus sits quite near your bladder, supported by the same group of ligaments and muscles. When the uterus is removed, there's a risk that local muscles and nerves could be damaged—and the ones closest by are the ones that affect your urinary tract. Any injury to those muscles or nerves can bring on incontinence.

In addition to these, a 2006 study found that Type 2 diabetes increases your chances of developing UI by up to 70%. Researchers discovered that lifestyle modifications for women with prediabetes (a condition where your blood-sugar numbers fall somewhere between normal and full-blown diabetes levels) could cut down that risk substantially. By losing some weight—less than 10 pounds, on average—you can knock down the risk of developing Type 2 diabetes and improve your bladder control all at once.

Your Treatment Options

When it comes to OAB and UI, you have a long menu of treatments to choose from. On the more traditional side, there are some prescription medications that can help with muscle control; relatively minor surgeries (for causes like an enlarged prostate); and some physical interventions (like catheters). For my patients, I like to start with the safest, least invasive approaches, and that often includes complementary and alternative treatments. These scientific approaches add a number of treatment options like:

- bladder training (to help you establish a more regular voiding pattern)
- Kegel exercises
- electrical stimulation
- herbal remedies
- dietary changes

Here we'll talk more about some of your better options, from how they work to potential side effects.

Prescription Medications

There are times when incontinence can be reversed with medicine alone. More often, though, the drug will be used in connection with a complementary technique (like Kegel exercises or dietary changes, for example). We're not talking about simple antibiotics here, though they may be used to clear up a specific infection. Rather, these prescriptions can sometimes control the incontinence itself...sounds good, but the side effect trade-off can be pretty high.

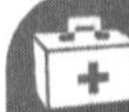

The Doctor Is In

Don't take antispasmodics if you have glaucoma, or at least avoid them unless you get the green light from your eye doctor. Antispasmodic drugs can make your condition worse, especially if you suffer from narrow-angle glaucoma. Here's why: These drugs can cause sudden increases in your eye pressure, even more than the glaucoma already does. Also, anyone with impaired kidney or liver function should stay away from these prescription medications.

The first class of incontinence medications are antispasmodics (also called anticholinergic agents). These drugs may be able to calm down an overactive bladder to help combat urge incontinence. Some of the more commonly prescribed brands include Detrol, Ditropan, Novartis, and Levsin. Side effects can include an extremely dry mouth (bad enough that it's hard to eat), constipation, cognition problems (like trouble remembering things), blurry vision, and dry eyes.

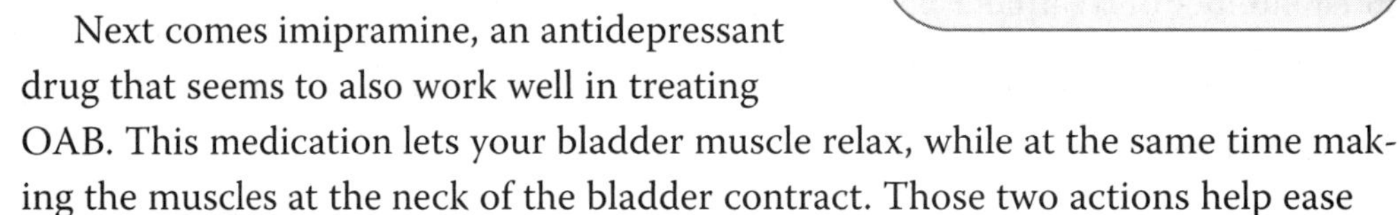

Next comes imipramine, an antidepressant drug that seems to also work well in treating OAB. This medication lets your bladder muscle relax, while at the same time making the muscles at the neck of the bladder contract. Those two actions help ease bladder filling and control emptying. Again, though, you can be hit with unwanted side effects when using this medication, like the abrupt lowering of your blood pressure as you move from sitting to standing, which can cause falls. Imipramine is also known to cause abnormal heartbeats in some people.

Along the same lines is duloxetine, originally an antidepressant and now being used to treat stress incontinence. While studies did show that the drug had some success in increasing the time between bathroom trips, that benefit also came with some side effects. The most common problem was nausea, severe enough for those affected patients to stop taking it. In one 2005 French study, researchers found 40 different adverse side effects of duloxetine and a high risk of interaction with other medications. These scientists concluded that the possible benefit—achievable without this medication—wasn't worth by the potential risks.

For women, some doctors suggest hormone-replacement therapy, as UI can be brought on by changing estrogen levels. This treatment, however, is known to cause potentially severe side effects, including increased risk of cancer and heart problems. On top of that, a 2005 study found that estrogen therapy could actually *increase* UI in postmenopausal women. Though many doctors will prescribe this course of action, I advise against it—especially since there are many other effective, much safer options you can try first.

Bladder Training

When you suffer from urge incontinence, timing is everything—and stretching out the time between urges can make a huge difference in your quality of life. One way to achieve this longer "safety" period is to retrain your bladder, which is a lot easier to do than you might think. This technique can take anywhere from two to 12 weeks to get your bladder on your preferred schedule; but once you get there, you can get back to your regular activities worry-free.

To retrain your bladder, you deliberately set a urination time table. Instead of waiting for an urge to strike, you go to the bathroom on your schedule—whether you feel like you need to or not. At first, the intervals between bathroom visits will be fairly short, about 30 minutes. From there, you will gradually lengthen the intervals in 30-minute increments until you get to three or four hours (whichever works better for your schedule and your body).

If you get the urge to urinate between scheduled bathroom breaks, try to resist by using one of the relaxation techniques described in chapter 8. Or you can try to do some Kegel exercises, if they help you keep that urge in check. Once the urge is gone, wait a full five minutes and then go to the bathroom, even if it's not the scheduled time yet, and even if you don't feel like you need to go anymore. If that five-minute wait gets easy, try stretching it to 10 minutes. Continue to stick to your schedule, even if the next visit seems unnecessary.

Kegel Exercises

Kegel exercises work especially well if you suffer from stress incontinence, as they help strengthen your bladder-control muscles. You can do these exercises any time, any place, and no one will be the wiser. Kegel exercises work equally well for men and women. But don't expect a quick fix here—this treatment method on its own can take up to three months to show results, but the improvement can be lasting.

It can be tough to get the hang of Kegel exercises at first, but stick with it. One of the easiest ways to conquer this move (especially for women) is to stop your urine flow midstream, without using your stomach or buttock muscles. Once you've got the motion down pat, squeeze those muscles for a count of 10, then relax for another 10-count. Repeat that squeeze 20 times and do three full sets of 20 each day, spread out over the course of the day. If you can't do the 10-second hold at first, start smaller (try a count of four or five) and work your way up to 10.

Men: Do It in Bed

Guys—if you're having a hard time finding the right muscles to do your Kegel exercises, try this while lying down. Act like you're trying to keep yourself from passing gas. When you squeeze those muscles, you may feel a pulling-type sensation. That feeling lets you know that you've found the right muscles. Once you've found them, you can start doing the exercises while standing or sitting, which ramps up the workout effect (like adding weight to your bench press). And remember to use ONLY these muscles when you're doing the Kegel exercises...clenching the wrong ones (like your buttock muscles) can actually put more pressure on the muscles controlling your bladder, which is exactly what you don't want.

Electrical Stimulation

Though it may sound shocking, electricity has been proven to help some people with OAB and UI. For quite some time now, people have been able to get electric stimulation to help the muscles at the floor of the pelvis work better. This electrical treatment is external and can be done right in the doctor's office. After several weeks of treatment, the effects of OAB and UI can be virtually wiped out for many sufferers.

One proven version of this treatment, called the NeoControl® Pelvic Floor Therapy System, was approved by the FDA in 1998. This nonsurgical therapy works by exercising pelvic-floor muscles through electrical pulsing and may restore their strength, endurance, and control. The therapy is pretty easy on patients: You just sit, fully clothed, in a special chair with electromagnets built into the seat...and NeoControl does the work for you. Basically, it helps your muscles do Kegel exercises while you sit back and relax.

Electrical-stimulation therapy appears to work especially well after radical prostatectomy—a Japanese study found the that Neocontrol method offered substantial UI reduction, with no reported side effects. It has also been successful for stress incontinence—a U.S. study found that women who'd never undergone continence surgery could achieve significant reduction of pad use, and some even enjoyed total dryness, after NeoControl therapy.

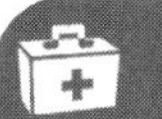

The Doctor Is In

Just like with drug dosages, different people can tolerate different levels of electrical stimulation. Expect some mild discomfort, at least at first, as the sensation feels unusual. For some people, though, the effect is more painful. So use caution if you have a low pain tolerance.

The therapy has shown enough success that an at-home kit has been developed, allowing you to perform this treatment on your own in the privacy of your own home. If you like to do things yourself, talk to your doctor about this more personal version of electrical-stimulation treatment. To provide the desired effect, your at-home unit will include an anal or vaginal electrode. Your doctor will instruct you on proper use and tell you precisely how long to treat yourself and how many treatments you'll need each day. Just like the doctor's-office version, this treatment typically takes several weeks to show optimal results.

If electrical stimulation sounds appealing but not the constant doctor visits (or self-imposed electrode use), you may want to consider an implant. This treatment is becoming more widely available in the United States, under the name of InterStim therapy. Though the device—also called a bladder pacemaker—has been FDA approved since 1999, it's just beginning to grow in popularity as an option for treating severe bladder problems. The mini machine sends small electrical pulses to your pelvic-floor muscles, and that seems to help with muscle strength and control. The implantation procedure takes place in two stages, allowing patient and doctor to make sure the device works as expected before implementing the more permanent second stage. In the first stage, the device is controlled by an external battery pack. Once everyone is happy with the results, a permanent pulse generator—similar to a cardiac pacemaker—is implanted to complete the second stage.

Statistics Depend on What You Read

More than 13 million Americans suffer from OAB or UI, according to medical statistics that is. But business statistics put that number as much higher. Why the big difference? Medical statistics are based on diagnosis and treatment, and sufferers often go without either. Business statistics are based on sales of products like Depend and Poise, best-selling adult-diaper brands most often used by sufferers who've avoided telling their doctors about what's really going on. In fact, sales of these products grew to about $1.2 billion in 2005—and that means the problem is a lot more common than most folks realize.

The Nutrition Factor

The dietary changes that best help with any kind of urinary problem start with a list of don'ts. For starters, try cutting out (or at least cutting down on) caffeine, alcohol, excess sugar, and sugar substitutes. Now add in some bacteria-fighting berries—cranberry and blueberry are best—to help you treat or prevent urinary tract infections that can make OAB and UI problems even worse. The high acidity of these fruits makes your urinary tract a very unfriendly environment for infection-causing micro-organisms. You can also try adding in some fermented dairy products, like yogurt and some cheeses, which also help keep bad bacteria at bay while boosting your supply of the gut-friendly kind.

There are also particular vitamins and minerals that can help keep things flowing normally:

- Vitamin C prevents bacteria from growing in your bladder. For the best results, take 1,000 mg of this beneficial nutrient three times each day.
- Zinc is a mineral well known for its immune-system-support properties. Add 30 mg per day to your regimen.
- A combination of calcium and magnesium can help improve

your muscle control and help you cut down on accidents. Take 500 mg of calcium and 250 mg of magnesium together twice a day. Magnesium works particularly well to fight urge incontinence.

- A big daily dose of betacarotene keeps your immune system sharp and can also keep your mucous membranes in optimal condition. Take up to 25,000 IU of betacarotene every day.

Remember, before you add any new supplements to your regimen, talk with a medical professional (like a licensed naturopath) to help determine the best starting dosage for you.

Herbal Solutions

Healing herbs can also provide long-term relief from the discomfort of incontinence. Whether you prefer to drink herbal tea or to take your herbs in capsule form, these natural remedies can help get your urinary tract back on track. Herbal remedies are often easier for your body to handle than prescription medications, rarely causing dangerous side effects. The trade-off is that they may take just a little bit longer to produce results—so don't expect an immediate, dramatic change in your symptoms. Most herbal remedies start to show results after about a week to 10 days, and total relief can take as long as six weeks. Stick with it, though, because once you see results, they'll be there to stay.

When it comes to dosage recommendations for these medicinal herbs, your own constitution is the most important guiding factor. To figure out the best herbal combinations and dosages for you, consider contacting a qualified herbalist or naturopath.

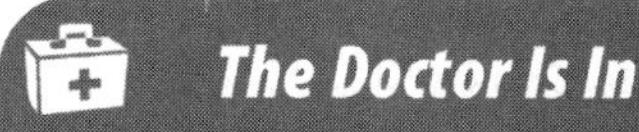

Most herbal remedies are safe for most people. There are, however, some people who should avoid certain herbs, and there are some herbs that can interact with prescription medications. Before you add any new herbs to your regimen, talk to your doctor or pharmacist.

Horsetail is one herb used for treating urinary problems successfully, in part due to its plentiful supply of easily absorbable silica—a mineral known to both maintain and strengthen tissue elasticity, making it a key member of your bladder-support team. You can make horsetail tea by adding one heaping tablespoon of the dried herb (readily available in health-food stores) to one cup of hot water—don't use boiling water for this tea. Let the tea steep for five to eight minutes along with a little sugar, which can help release more silica from the leaves. If drinking horsetail tea doesn't appeal to you, consider the capsule form. Start with 300 milligrams three times per day until your system gets used to the herb. If that's tolerable, you can increase to as much as the maximum safe dosage of 6 grams (that's 6,000 milligrams) per day—but spread that out over three doses as well. Do not use horsetail if you're already taking diuretics, unless your doctor says it's safe—the combination can cause excessive fluid loss, and that can lead to a serious electrolyte imbalance.

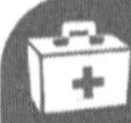

The Doctor Is In

Saw palmetto has been in the news recently, mostly in stories of doubt about its effectiveness. A lot of my patients swear by this herb—but I make sure they get the right variety. When you get saw palmetto, be sure to buy the fat-soluble variety, standardized to contain at least 85% fatty acids and sterols. (It should say that right on the bottle.)

For UI due to an enlarged prostate, an herb called stinging nettle has been shown to provide relief, especially when taken together with a partner herb called saw palmetto. Some studies indicate that this herbal combo may relieve a variety of urinary problems due to BPH—including reduced flow, incomplete bladder emptying, dripping, and constant urge. Both of these herbs are easily found at health-food stores. The easiest way to take stinging nettle is in capsule form (made of the dried leaves). Start with 2 grams three times per day. Once your system is used to the herb, you can safely take up to 4 grams three times per day. As for the saw palmetto, the recommended dosage for BPH is 320 milligrams of standardized extract per day. You can take that all at once or split it into two doses; both ways have been proven equally effective.

Another herbal option is marshmallow root, though this one is best taken as a cold infusion. To make up a batch, put one heaping teaspoon of marshmallow root (available at most health-food stores) into one quart of cold water. Let that mixture steep overnight, and then strain it in the morning. Drink your cold marshmallow root tea throughout the day. This concoction has anti-inflammatory and tissue-soothing properties, both of which may ease your UI symptoms.

In and Out

Here's a surprising connection for you: Folks suffering from constipation may find themselves developing UI. Turns out that straining to pass hard stool out can actually make it harder to keep urine in. That's because bearing down to move stool along may weaken the nerves in charge of keeping your bladder's filling and emptying under control. Luckily, there are some simple solutions that can treat constipation and help prevent UI. Boosting your daily fiber intake will help, and you can get that in some pretty delicious ways—baked apples, bran muffins (even better with raisins), or a cup of hot coffee first thing in the morning (even decaf will do). Or you can try some beneficial herbs, like a tea made out of senna, one of the world's safest and most effective laxatives. You can cook up an infusion of this tea by placing six to 10 senna pods in a cup of boiling water, and then letting the mixture steep for at least 10 minutes. Strain the liquid into a drinking cup and sip it at night on an empty stomach; by morning, your bowels will be raring to go.

CHAPTER 5

Banishing Aches and Pains

Look around you: There's a pill for everything...and when it comes to pain, you have dozens of pills to choose from. Problem is, lots of these pills—and not just the prescription ones—come with a long list of nasty, sometimes deadly, side effects. Sure, they can make your pain go away, at least for a little while, but is four hours of relief really worth the risk of lifelong consequences?

Because there are so many readily available commercial painkillers, we forget that people used to rely on nature to relieve their aches and pains. Before there were drug stores on every corner and on-line pharmacies that could ship orders for next-day delivery, people turned to whatever remedy was right in front of them...like feverfew to relieve headache pain or alfalfa tea to ease arthritis. (I'll talk more about both of these in a moment).

Most of the medical professionals you'll run into these days turn their noses up at "old-fashioned folk remedies." But science is proving them wrong. More and more research is proving that these time-tested pain relievers work—often as well as or better than commercial painkillers—without inflicting side effects that are just as bad as the pain was.

There are literally dozens of natural ways to treat your pain, whatever the cause, wherever the ache. Even better, many of these remarkable remedies do more than just temporarily relieve pain—they fix the underlying problem, so you can remain pain-free for the long haul.

From foods to herbs to specially designed exercises to some pretty fancy new high-tech solutions, you'll be able to find relief for virtually any pain that strikes you.

The Diet Solution to a Pain-Free Life

Believe it or not, what you eat can impact how much pain you're in. Just adding a few foods to your daily diet can noticeably reduce pain and inflammation...and eating them regularly can prevent the pain from coming back. Add to those some herbal teas—each of which can ease specific aches on its own—and you can help your body fight aches and pains. Add some special spices, and you can increase the pain-fighting powers in any meal. And adding some specific supplements to your regimen may just keep your pain at bay all the time.

> **Beware the Nightshade**
>
> Got stiff joints...pain...inflammation? The reason could be no farther away than the food on your plate, because some foods can actually cause these symptoms. And when you stop eating them, your symptoms could literally disappear, almost overnight.
>
> If you're in pain, try avoiding these foods for a couple of weeks and see how much better you feel. The "Don't Eat" list includes potatoes, tomatoes, eggplant, pepper (every kind, from chilies to bells to the kind you sprinkle on your food). Remember, any form of these veggies can add to the problem, so no fries with ketchup, no chips and salsa, and no eggplant parmesan.

Fight Pain With Food

You probably know that every natural food contains some healthful compounds—vitamins, minerals, antioxidants. Well, some of those compounds also have anti-inflammatory properties, others have cell-strengthening properties, and still others have analgesic properties. Eating these foods, especially when they're topped off with particular herbs and spices (as you'll see below), can eliminate your pain safely and effectively, without an expensive trip to the drug store.

Along with each food listed below, you'll find the kind of pain it's best at fighting. If you've got more than one kind of pain—headaches and arthritis, for example—you can safely mix any of these foods, unlike medications, which can have deadly interactions when taken together.

Black beans: Got back pain? Think black beans. One centuries-old Asian remedy for back pain is to eat just 2 tablespoons of black beans every day for a month. Back pain is often the result of poor tone in the muscles that support the spinal column...and black beans make great protein, crucial for maintaining muscle strength.

Celery: Inflammation is a major pain causer, and celery is a diuretic, which reduces excess fluid build-up. That, in turn, can reduce the inflammation associated with arthritis, along with the pain. The Japanese believe strongly in the pain-relieving effects of celery: They recommend eating cooked or raw celery daily for one to two months...or you could substitute a daily glass of celery juice.

Honey: Honey, which has natural pain-relieving powers, is a traditional Chinese remedy for headaches. Find 100% raw honey and eat it straight out of the jar. Or you can mix three large spoonfuls of it in boiled water and drink up. You can spike your honey with buckthorn berries, licorice, cinnamon, mint leaves, and orange peels, all also used to ease throbbing heads. **Doctor's Orders:** *Stay away from honey if you have low or high blood sugar.*

Cherries: To get rid of arthritis pain, the Japanese eat six to eight cherries a day (canned, frozen, or fresh—any form will do). Cherries contain magnesium, a natural painkiller, and potassium, which acts as a diuretic. This remedy works particularly well for gout sufferers.

Strawberries: A Swiss botanist made a case for strawberries as a remedy for rheumatism after a steady diet of them helped relieve his own joint pain—probably because strawberries help eliminate uric acid from the system. When

The One-Cent Solution

Some researchers believe that a low-copper diet may cause headaches in susceptible people. The theory is that a copper deficiency makes the blood-vessel walls constrict and cause pain. Good food sources of copper include oysters, lobster, liver, nuts, seeds, green olives, and wheat bran.

uric acid builds up, it can crystallize in your joints, causing some serious pain.

Papaya: Natives of the Fiji Islands were the first to recognize the papaya's powerful curative abilities. Research is being conducted to develop the fruit's active enzyme, papain, to treat herniated (slipped) discs in the lower area of the back, a frequent source of severe back pain. For now, just visit the produce aisle and grab some papayas—they make great smoothies year-round.

A Cup of Pain Relief

Lots of people believe in the restorative powers of a warm cup of tea (I prefer the iced version myself). But when it comes to relieving pain, any temperature will do, whichever way you can drink it faster. On top of their unique tastes, each tea serves up a particular pain-fighting remedy. For extra pain-fighting abilities, sweeten your tea with honey (unless you have any kind of blood-sugar problem).

Blackstrap molasses: The British swear by crude blackstrap molasses dissolved in water for pain relief—I gave it a try, and it really worked. When you take it every morning, this preparation appears to ease and even eliminate joint pain. That may be because molasses is an excellent source of minerals, including potassium and magnesium. You can find it in any grocery store, usually in the baking section or near the honey.

Black currant: A rheumatism remedy that is very popular in Europe—especially among the mountain people of eastern Europe—is black currant tea. They brew a tea from the leaves of the black currant bush. You can avoid trekking through the meadows by just buying prebagged black currant tea at any health-food store.

Cowslip: Cowslip, which grows wild in nearly all pastures and meadows, is a gentle pain reliever—and also a good source of natural aspirin. A tea made of cowslip petals, honey, sugar, and lemon juice is a tasty treatment for headaches. Cowslip can be bought in cut or powdered form through most mail-order herb companies and health-food stores.

Ginger: Fresh ginger tea is used throughout the world to treat headaches (among other ailments). You can make it by grating and squeezing gingerroot to extract the juice. Then add about a teaspoon of the juice to a cup of hot water.

Mint: Spearmint is an antispasmodic and a diuretic, making it great for pain relief—especially when that pain comes with cramping. You can get your spearmint in pretty much any form, but the tea is particularly soothing.

Alfalfa: Alfalfa tea is well known for its anti-inflammatory properties. Because it reduces knuckle swelling and joint pain, alfalfa is often recommended for people who spend a lot of time using their hands—like for typing or knitting. Drink a cup of alfalfa tea several times throughout the day. For headaches, try alfalfa seed tea for fast and effective pain relief.

Chinese angelica/Dong quai: A Chinese version of angelica, called dong quai, is used by lots of herbalists I know to relieve headaches. Make a medicinal tea by boiling one large slice of dried dong quai root in 2 cups of water, uncovered, for about 10 minutes. Remove the root (save it—you can use it again) and then sip the liquid. You can find dong quai in Asian markets and many health-food stores.

Chrysanthemum: In India and China, tension headaches are commonly soothed by a tea made from dried yellow chrysanthemum. Prepackaged tea bags are available in most health-food stores. This tea tastes much better with some sweetener added.

A Spicy Solution

You can spice up ordinary meals and eliminate your pain in one fell swoop by using these savory seasonings. They work powerfully alone and even more impressively together.

Cayenne pepper: This steaming-hot seasoning contains capsaicin, a natural anti-inflammatory. Heap it on foods by the teaspoon for hours of pain relief.

Garlic: Because of its natural ability to reduce inflammation, garlic can ward off the pain and discomfort felt by arthritis sufferers—just three or four cloves a day can do the trick.

Ginger: Ginger is highly effective for treating both osteoarthritis and rheumatoid arthritis. Because it increases blood circulation, ginger carries inflammatory substances away from your aching joints.

Supplements to Stop the Pain

When pain is an everyday issue, it calls for an everyday solution. And when it comes to pain, I'll take prevention over relief any day. When you add these supplements into your regimen, you're taking steps to rid your life of constant pain. Unlike most medications, these take some time to work, anywhere from several days to several months. But when they start working, they can actually fix the problem instead of just covering it up, and you will notice the difference every single day.

Glucosamine. This supplement got a lot of press over the past few years, often times in connection with chondroitin (which I generally avoid recommending). Some reports said it worked great, others said it did nothing. But I've seen it work wonders—virtually erasing joint pain. An elderly gentleman came to see me for help with debilitating arthritic knee-joint pain. Now this was a man whose goal in life was to continue grubbing around on his hands and knees in his garden. (He actually finds weeding enjoyable!) So I started him on straight glucosamine sulfate and told him to give it a whole month before expecting results...and in well under one month, he came back to show me that crawling around was no longer a problem at all. Try taking 1 gram of glucosamine sulfate twice a day, away from food (meaning at least one hour before or two hours after eating). You can take it with water or juice, but avoid taking it with any kind of protein (like milk).

Vitamin B6. This nutrient can successfully treat moderate cases of carpal tunnel syndrome and also act as a preventive. Researchers from the Kaiser Permanente Medical Center in Hayward, California successfully treated CTS patients with 200 mg per day of vitamin B6, administered over a period of three months. I've seen it work. Back in the days when I was the company doctor for AT&T, lots of folks had this problem. I'd put them on B6, which works even better when taken along with 500 mg of magnesium daily. Within just 90 days, the pain would be gone for good. How does it work? Carpal tunnel syndrome causes a reduction in the rate at which nerve impulses travel, and B6 therapy seems to speed up the nerve impulses to the hand—reducing the pressure and pain.

Calcium. Calcium is an important supplement even for people who don't get migraines. It is best taken at night, because it also has a calming effect on the body and helps promote sleep. That same calming effect helps migraine sufferers by relaxing muscles in the head and easing tightening in the temples.

Chromium. If you suffer from low blood sugar or hypoglycemia, you are a likely candidate for a migraine, and a chromium supplement may help you by regulating your blood-sugar levels.

Feverfew. This member of the daisy family has been used extensively in Europe to treat migraines, and studies in both Europe and the United States. have shown that this herb unquestionably relieves the pain. My best results with it have actually been with non-migraine headaches, but I've seen it work for both types. Feverfew contains an anti-inflammatory agent that helps dilate the tight, constricted blood vessels that are characteristic of migraines. It also contains a compound that stops blood-vessel spasms from occurring. Feverfew is most effective if taken in capsule from every day as a preventive...but you can still use it during a flare-up for quick relief if you take it at the first sign of trouble. To boost the power, take it along with magnesium—that helps it work even faster and has gotten me more surprised thank-you calls than I can count.

D Is for Pain

Lots of folks with chronic pain are misdiagnosed, as doctors stick to comfortable diagnoses like fibromyalgia and stress as the culprits. But with a little more work on their parts—one simple blood test—they could learn that the real problem is a Vitamin D deficiency. In fact, one study of patients with unexplained pain found that 93% of them were lacking that essential nutrient. If you suffer from bone and muscle pain and no one can figure out why, ask your doctor to test your Vitamin D blood levels.

Fish oils. Fish oils, especially those from fatty fish (herring, salmon, mackerel, tuna, and sardines) are good sources of omega-3 fatty acids. These fatty acids interfere with the formation of prostaglandins that can lead to inflammation. A daily serving of fresh fish (or fish oil capsules if you don't like fish or are concerned about the high mercury content) can produce noticeable results.

Potassium. This important mineral is found in many common fruits and vegetables. So when you're achy or sore, increase your consumption of bananas, which have one of the highest potassium levels of all foods. Other good food sources of potassium include cantaloupes, oranges, avocados, raw spinach, raw cabbage, and raw celery.

Niacin. A member of the B-vitamin family, niacin helps promote blood flow and can minimize muscle cramping. Start with small quantities—less than 250 mg per day—and be sure to take it with food to avoid possible side effects like flushing and itchy skin.

Better Than Glucosamine

You can start looking on the drugstore shelves for JointVital, the U.S. trade name for a Danish product called LitoZin. Though many are comparing it to glucosamine, it doesn't work the same way...and some studies have shown that it relieves joint pain more effectively. JointVital fights inflammation *and* rebuilds cartilage, getting to the source of pain. One study found that this preparation worked in 82% of patients (compared with just 40% for glucosamine)...and completely removed the need for "rescue pills" like NSAIDs.

Stretch, Strengthen, and Stop Aching

Your body feels different kinds of pain in different ways, and each kind affects distinct areas and movements. Contrary to what most people think, chronic pain is best managed with movement—even though that seems like the opposite of what you should do. Special exercises can help your body fight pain more effectively, and keep that pain from coming back.

Here's the caution: Don't overdo it. Start slowly and move slowly. It may be uncomfortable at first, but it shouldn't make you hurt more.

Exercise Arthritis Pain Away

To combat arthritis effectively, you need the full circle of exercises: flexibility, strength, and endurance. Don't do it all at once—you can rotate days. Start with very light weights, 2 pounds or less, and short spurts of weight-bearing exercise (like walking). If lifting light weights or walking is too difficult to start out with, you can try some of these gentler exercises to help you gain a better range of mobility. For example:

- If you have arthritis in your lower body, get into a heated pool as often as you can, every day if possible. Then walk back and forth across the shallow end until you start getting tired.
- For arthritis flare-ups in your hands, squeeze a soft rubber ball. You can also twist a large rubber band, and gently spread the fingers apart, using the rubber band as resistance. Or exercise your hands in the sink or in a pot of warm water.
- Yoga seems to be especially effective in treating arthritis. You can find classes at local community centers and even some hospitals. You can also try do-it-yourself tapes or DVDs, if you prefer to practice yoga at home—but go to at least a couple of classes led by a qualified instructor first. The poses can be hard to do at first, at least to do properly, and if you do them wrong, you could end up in more pain than before.

When you're ready to take things up a notch, give these arthritis-banishing exercises a shot:

The Shoulder Turn

This exercise can improve the movement in your shoulders. Start with your hands locked behind your neck, elbows pointing straight in front of you. Slowly bring your elbows out sideways as far as you can and hold for five seconds. Then bring them together and hold for five seconds. Repeat.

The Toe-Heel Lift

Here's a way to keep your ankles flexible, which can make walking more comfortable. Sit in a chair with your feet flat on the floor. Keeping your heels on the floor, raise your toes and the front of your feet as high as you can (your toes should now be pointing up). Move your feet to the right. Then bring your toes back to the floor and raise your heels as high as you can. Lower your heels back down to the floor and then repeat the same movements to the left. Then repeat the whole cycle from the beginning.

The Hip and Knee Bend

Do this exercise to maintain strength and motion in your swollen knees and hips. Lie on your back, knees bent with your feet flat on the floor. Bring one leg up and grab it behind the thigh, pulling it toward you. Hold that position for five seconds. Slowly return to the starting position and repeat the same movements with your other leg. Then repeat the whole cycle from the beginning.

Exercise Your Back Pain Away

Everyone hurts his back from time to time—it's almost guaranteed to happen at some point. What's uncertain is where (on your back) you'll have pain and how much pain you'll feel. The answers determine the right treatment, and the right preventive measures once the initial pain is dealt with.

The vast majority of back problems are caused by muscle or ligament strain. Those kinds are temporary in nature and somewhat easier to deal with (treatment-wise, that is). That means you can both fix this problem and prevent future pain if you're willing to spend a few minutes exercising every day. It works like this: The inflammation that brings on your pain can be caused by noxious chemicals released by damaged cells. Better blood circulation carries those toxins out with the rest of the waste...so any therapy that moves muscles and causes increased blood flow speeds recovery.

If you already have a chronic back problem (the kind that never really leaves and flares up from time to time), you need to improve your strength and flexibility in order to see a real change. Concentrate on your lower back, both

Prevent Cramps

The most common reason for cramping is muscle fatigue combined with an imbalance of salt and water in the body. That is why athletes drink plenty of water and sports drinks like Gatorade, which help restore proper levels of salt (and other minerals) to the body. For a natural (and much less sugary than Gatorade) fix, try Recharge, available in the natural-foods section of your grocery store.

when it's extended (straight) and when it's flexed (bent). And don't neglect your hamstrings and your stomach muscles.

Here are a few exercises you can easily do to prevent back injuries or pain:

Cat stretch: Get on all fours, with your back level. Slowly arch your back so you look like a cat (your head will drop, and your mid-back will rise). Hold that position for a count of 2. Repeat the exercise five to 10 times.

Mid-back stretch: Kneel on the floor. Extend your arms and torso forward, reaching as far as you can. Hold for a count of 10. Then repeat the stretch three times.

Hamstring stretch: Lie on your back. Bend your leg and bring your knee toward your chest, supporting the back of your thigh with your hands behind your knee. Attempt to straighten your knee until a comfortable stretch is felt on the back of your thigh. Hold for a count of 10 to 15. Repeat with the opposite leg. Then repeat the entire cycle two to five times.

The Proof Is in the Position

Viniyoga, an easy-to-learn style of the ancient exercise, has found its way into the medical journals. A groundbreaking new study shows that it may reduce chronic back pain (along with the need for potentially harmful painkillers) and even improve how well your back functions.

Researchers worked with 101 patients, all with chronic lower-back pain. The patients were split into three groups: One practiced yoga, one attended traditional exercise classes, and one received a book about back pain. At the 26-week mark, only 21 percent of the yoga group still needed pain drugs, compared with 50 percent of the other exercise group and 59 percent of the book group.

Single knee-to-chest stretch: Lie on the floor on your back and pull one knee into your chest until a comfortable stretch is felt in your lower back and buttocks. Hold that position for a 10 to 15 count. Then switch to the opposite knee. Repeat the entire cycle two to five times.

Double knee to chest stretch: Lie on your back. Pull both knees to your chest until you feel a comfortable stretch in your lower back. Hold for a 10 to 15 count. Repeat the stretch two to five times.

Other exercises, like yoga and tai chi, can also help strengthen and stretch back muscles. In Hong Kong, back pain is treated not only by doctors but also by masters of kung fu. The concentrated exercises and controlled body movements required to practice this martial art effectively treats most forms of back pain.

Exercise for Carpal Tunnel Syndrome

Lots of folks think this isn't a "real" condition—but it is, and it is mighty painful. Anyone who uses a lot of fine finger movements is at risk—people who type a lot, play the piano, or do needlework, for example. Once it strikes, you have to give your hands a break from the regular routine or risk making your condition worse. To speed your recovery, try these exercises—you can literally do them anywhere.

For treatment: Move your hands around in gentle circles for a few minutes about four times a day. This rotation of the wrists restores circulation and eliminates a major cause of CTS symptoms.

For prevention: If you don't have symptoms (at least not yet) but your daily activities make you a likely candidate, try this preventive workout: With a rubber band around your fingers, open and close them 10 times, two or three times a day. Increase the number of repetitions and the tension on the rubber band as you gain strength in your fingers.

Alternative Solutions Offer Remarkable Relief

More and more patients have been shying away from conventional medicine—which usually involves expensive trips to specialists and pillboxes full of prescriptions—and coming to me for true solutions to their pain problems. I'm all for medicine when it's called for...but for pain, especially chronic pain, treatments outside the mainstream just plain work better. I don't

Fantasy Fights Pain

Love may conquer all, but romantic fantasies can wipe out pain. A study from Johns Hopkins University found that thinking steamy thoughts could combat pain...not to mention dimming anxiety to make you less tense. Just think about a pleasurable romantic encounter—your honeymoon, a first kiss, even a candlelight dinner—and see your pain fade into the background.

mean only that they let you feel better right away, though many of these methods do just that, but also that they make a difference in your everyday life by eliminating and treating the sources of your pain.

Relaxation

Stress can cause physical pain, and vice versa. When the two team up and you're hit with both pain and tension, they can be hard to overcome—your muscles clench, your blood pressure rises, and your breathing becomes more shallow. And the more people tell you to relax, the more tense you may get. But that's what I'm going to tell you—because relaxation can reverse the effects of both stress and physical pain.

Therapeutic relaxing is different than kicking back in front of the tube with a beer or a glass of wine. It involves concentration and focus, more of an active relaxation. These techniques can help you calm yourself down, in body and mind, letting you get back the control and move that pain right out of your body. You can find detailed instructions for several relaxation techniques in Chapter 8.

Relaxation Kicks Post-Op Pain

Surgery hurts—when you wake up after the fact, there will be pain. People know that, they expect it, and that can make the pain feel even worse. But a remarkable study found that relaxation and music can substantially cut back on post-op pain. Out of 500 patients, the groups that listened to music, practiced relaxation, or both reported considerably less pain—as proven by how much less frequently they pressed the buttons on their painkiller pumps.

Acupuncture

If you've never tried it, the thought of relieving pain by being stuck with needles may sound ridiculous—but there are centuries of practice and lots of new science that say it really does the trick...painlessly and effectively.

The proof is in the numbers:

- A large German trial (involving over 1,000 participants, all with knee osteoarthritis) found that just 10 sessions of acupuncture resulted in at least a 36% improvement for 53% of the patients who got it.

- Another German study, this one looking into the effectiveness of acupuncture for chronic lower-back pain, found that pain and quality-of-life measures improved by up to 75% with acupuncture...and this study included 11,630 patients.
- Yet another large German study (of 14,161 patients with chronic neck pain) found that treatment with acupuncture improved pain and disability symptoms by 16.2% in just three months, compared with just a 3.9% improvement for the control group.
- A team of researchers conducted an analysis of 10 separate trials testing the effectiveness of acupuncture for chronic neck pain. Their conclusion: overall, patients who received acupuncture reported less pain both immediately and at short-term follow-up.

And here's another interesting statistic for you: Around 15 million Americans have tried acupuncture with much success, so much so that many insurance companies will cover the treatments—making even the payments less painful.

Hydrotherapy

Hydrotherapy sounds high-tech, but it really just means soaking in water. You may already use this method all the time: taking a hot shower when your shoulders are sore...soaking tired-out muscles in the bath...sticking your aching feet into a foot bath. Sometimes, though, treating one area of the body actually helps another.

In the Orient, people with severe back pain soak their feet in hot water for 20 to 30 minutes. Back pain and spasms can both be relieved in this way. That's because the nerves that go to the feet come off the lower spinal column, and warming them may do the trick to soothe your aching back. CAUTION: *If you have ulcers, avoid this treatment. It may stimulate blood circulation, which could indirectly trigger acid secretion in the stomach.*

Rub It In

Topical pain relievers can feel miraculous—they work fast and last long. Since you'll know almost right away if the pain stops, you can quickly figure out which rub works best for your condition. Don't use more than one at a time—in fact, to be on the safe side, don't use more than one formula per day on the same spot, as different compounds may interact with each other and cause unpleasant effects (like itching). And always wash your hands with soap after an application—just a drop in your eye or nose can bring on a new (and really bad) kind of pain.

Arnica: Used topically, arnica can soothe sore muscles when rubbed directly on the area in pain. You can buy prepared gels and lotions at almost any grocery store and many pharmacies—gels work faster.

Chinese tiger balm: Chinese tiger balm is a healing ointment that contains aromatic oils of camphor, menthol, peppermint, clove, and cajeput. Massage it into any painful area (except a bruise), and it increases blood flow to surface skin...making your pain a thing of the past.

Lavender: Lavender is a natural sedative, analgesic, and antispasmodic, providing three ways to conquer headache pain all in one tidy little package. Make yourself a soothing rub of one part lavender oil mixed with two parts olive oil and massage it on your throbbing temples.

Camphor: Italians combine equal parts of olive oil and camphor and rub it in to the sore area. This simple home remedy is the basis for many over-the-counter preparations available in the United States (like Chinese tiger balm). Camphor works by increasing blood circulation to the skin.

There's a Reason They're Called Pain KILLERS

Everyone pops painkillers from time to time, yours truly included. Heck, I even prescribe them for patients with serious pain...but with extreme caution, and for very short times. The truth is that virtually all commercial painkillers pose some danger, even the ones that seem totally harmless.

Like acetaminophen (a.k.a. Tylenol), which can trigger deadly liver damage. Or NSAIDs, including Cox-2 inhibitors, which can cause heart attacks...especially in folks who have already had heart attacks.

Cayenne pepper: A cayenne pepper rub is a great external treatment for muscle injuries but works best on chronic pain (like arthritis). Capsaicin, the active chemical in these peppers, relieves pain when applied to the skin. Capsaicin affects the sensory nerve and stimulates blood flow to the area, which reduces inflammation. You can find premixed preparations at the health-food store or at regular pharmacies under the brand name Zostrix. Whether you get the brand-name version or the generic one (just called capsaicin cream), go for the .075% strength. Cayenne can take a day or two to start working, but keep at it and you'll feel it kick in. One word of caution: After use, wash your hands VERY WELL—and keep your hands away from your face or any open wounds. Take my advice, as someone who's been in a hurry after applying capsaicin cream and paid the price (yes, I use this all the time): This stuff is HOT, and it will burn eyes and noses on contact.

What's the WOMAC Scale?

When it comes to studying osteoarthritis pain, researchers had to come up with a universal measurement. Meet the Western Ontario and McMaster (WOMAC) universities' solution. The WOMAC scale combines scores for pain level (0 through 20), physical function (0 through 68), and stiffness (0 through 8) to come up with an overall pain index for study participants.

So when you read that pain was improved by 32% or 51%, that shows how much better the patient felt according to his "before and after" WOMAC scores.

Comfrey: Comfrey leaves can speed up the healing process for sprains and strains. Boil about 8 ounces of it in a small amount of water for about five minutes. Once it's cool enough to touch, put the whole thing—leaves and all—in a soft cloth and apply to your injury. For larger or more serious sprains, wrap the wounded area with a compress made only with the comfrey liquid. Simply boil the leaves (a couple of ounces should be enough for each application) in 3/4 pint of water for 20 minutes. Strain and use the water to saturate a large, soft cloth. Leave the cloth on your injury until the compress cools. Then remove and replace with a fresh one.

Ginger: In Japan, they use ginger to heal aching muscles and relieve tightness by making ginger oil and applying it directly to the sore area. Just grate some fresh ginger root and squeeze the juice into a bowl. Mix with an equal amount of olive oil and massage into the skin. Many Asians also use ginger in their baths. To try that, grate about 1 teaspoon of fresh ginger and squeeze the juice directly into your bath water. Soak until the water cools. This remedy also works very well for muscle cramps.

The High-Tech Track

Every day, inventors and researchers come up with new or improved ways to fight pain. Some of their innovations come in the form of stronger pain pills—but those often come with bigger side-effect consequences. Others look at new techniques that seem to interrupt pain feelings, or at least make them easier to deal with.

Millimeter Wave Therapy

One of the latest pain therapy techniques is still in the pilot-study phases, but is showing incredible promise. It's called millimeter wave therapy (MWT), and it works by applying low-intensity electromagnetic millimeter waves to your body from a very close range. The technique has been used to treat numerous types of pain, from headaches to joint pain to post-op pain to neuropathic (nerve) pain—all with some success.

Like for osteoarthritis patients: In this study, some patients received MWT in addition to regular pain meds while others got only their pills. The patients who got MWT had ten sessions, each twenty minutes long, reported feeling better after just two or three sessions. The scientists also found that pain intensity was measurably reduced, joint mobility greatly improved, and lower levels of C-reactive protein (which is a measure of inflammation).

Bioelectric Therapy

Along the same lines as MWT, bioelectric therapy offers a safe, drug-free way to get rid of pain. This method literally blocks pain messages to your brain and encourages your body to produce endorphins—its natural pain relievers. This treatment holds off pain temporarily, rather than on a permanent basis, but it makes a great addition to your overall pain-management program. In fact, folks who've tried this were able to cut back on pain meds by up to 50%!

This treatment method has shown success for treating a wide range of pain conditions, like:

- back pain
- migraines
- muscle pain
- arthritis
- diabetic neuropathy (a kind of nerve pain commonly felt by diabetics)
- TMJ (joint pain that hits you in the jaw)

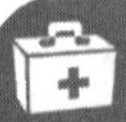

The Doctor Is In

Stay away from bioelectric treatment methods if you have a pacemaker or have blood clots in your arms or legs. You should also avoid getting treated if you're suffering from a current bacterial infection—colds and flu don't count (they're viruses).

Revitalize Your Get-Up-and-Go

Almost everyone expects to slow down as he gets older—but that doesn't have to be the case. You've heard the stories about 81-year-old trapeze artists...73-year-old deep-sea divers...86-year-old marathon runners. Those people don't have to be the surprising few. All of us can have virtually boundless energy if we just supply our bodies with what they need.

With some modest diet and exercise changes, you can have as much energy as you did 20 years ago. Walking to the store will be energizing instead of energy-sapping. Playing with your grandkids won't wear you out in 10 minutes. And the more you do, the more you'll be able to do...and the more energetic you'll feel.

Safe Energy Supplements

There's certainly no lack of energy supplements on the market, many claiming the power to instantly revitalize you. They may contain heavy doses of caffeine and other known stimulants...and they will rev you up, at least for the moment. The problem is that unless you keep taking them, you'll crash—and may feel even more tired than you did before.

On the safe and natural side, there are plenty of quick, temporary pick-me-ups to help get you going when your energy just drops off. For a longer-term solution to constant fatigue, different supplements are called for...the ones that support crucial body functions and let you tap into your body's natural energy supply.

The Quick-Fix Gang

There are a lot of natural stimulants you can use when you need a quick energy boost. These fatigue busters are very safe, as long as you use them properly. They will perk you up, pretty quickly, but the effects will be short-lived. Use these to combat sudden dips in energy, but not as a way to battle long-term chronic fatigue.

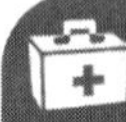

The Doctor Is In

For some folks, even natural stimulants are not safe. If you've been having heart troubles or have been diagnosed with high blood pressure, these stimulants are not for you. Also, some of these remedies may interact with prescription drugs—so if you're taking any medications at all, talk to your doctor or pharmacist before you use one of these pick-me-ups.

Ginseng may be the best-known herb used in traditional Chinese medicine—and for good reason. Studies have shown that it has energy-producing capabilities and can even help your body process oxygen more efficiently...which also helps boost energy and stamina. This herb has two distinct forms, Panax and Siberian. Both are used to increase energy levels, and the Siberian form also offers particular compounds that fight fatigue. You can take up to 650 mg of Panax ginseng or up to 300 mg of Siberian ginseng twice a day (for either). You can take these supplements with or without food.

Gotu kola has been used by the Chinese for centuries as an energy tonic. Gotu kola isn't even remotely related to Coca-Cola, or any cola beverage for that matter, despite the sound of its name...but it can give you a quick alertness jolt. You can find this lesser-known herbal pick-me-up in a ready-made tonic, in capsule form, and in a powder that you can make into tea. If you try the capsules, take 200 mg (of the freeze-dried herb) up to three times per day.

Peppermint acts quickly to restore energy and combat fatigue. Long-distance truckers rely on this natural herb to keep them alert during those long hauls across the country. You can chew on sprigs of fresh peppermint or peppermint gum or simply take a whiff of peppermint oil to help keep you awake and alert.

Yerba mate is the national beverage of Paraguay, and it's been called "the ideal stimulant." The tasty tea-like beverage does offer a caffeine kick but is much gentler than regular American coffee or tea.

The Energy Foundation

Just like your DVD player relies on electricity to power it up, your body relies on a special mix of nutrients to provide its power source. Some nutrients work in energy production, others in metabolism, and still others in distribution...but you need all of them, working together to adequately supply your body with the fuel it needs to just keep going.

Here are the main players in this nutritional line up:

- B vitamins, especially B12
- chromium
- iron
- magnesium
- manganese
- amino acids
- essential fatty acids

Let's start with the **B vitamins**, which often come together in a single B-complex formula. These nutrients are must-haves for healthy nervous and immune systems...and they're usually the first to go when we're not getting enough nutrition from food. As we get older, our bodies may absorb less of these vitamins from food...and that can make us feel plain old tired. A good B-complex supplement can turn that around. The best ones contain 50 micrograms of B12, 400 micrograms of folic acid, and 50 micrograms of each of the other B vitamins. Take your B-complex supplement every morning with your breakfast.

Your body needs **chromium** to help it utilize the sugars in the foods you eat. Most people don't get nearly enough of this trace mineral, and that's especially true of folks with diabetes. You see, chromium affects how your body regulates its blood-sugar and insulin levels...and when those are out of whack, you can be socked with chronic fatigue. There are a few different types of chromium supplements, but the ones I recommend most are chromium picolinate and chromium-enriched yeast (also called GTF-chromium). Either way, the dose is 200 micrograms per day, best taken with food. The enriched yeast is the most natural form (which moves it to the top of the list in my book) and rarely a problem even for people with yeast sensitivities.

Iron gets the oxygen moving through your body and helps with energy production. When your iron supplies run low, weakness and fatigue will set in, and that can make it harder to concentrate. Iron is a tricky supplement, though, because your body holds on to it tightly. That can lead to too much iron in your system, and that condition comes with its own set of consequences (constipation, for example). It's a good idea to get an iron test before you start supplementing and to talk with your doctor about getting the right dosage. To prevent deficiency, men can safely take up to 10 mg per day and women can take up to 15 mg per day. Other good sources of iron include calves liver and dessicated liver tablets.

If you've been fatigued for quite a while, a **magnesium** deficiency may very well be to blame. Most people don't get enough of this essential mineral, and most mainstream doctors don't measure levels. But magnesium is a crucial component for manufacturing the actual energy source (adenosine triphosphate, or ATP) that's inside every cell. Without enough magnesium, your cells just can't make enough energy. It takes about a month to rebuild magnesium stores, so don't expect instant results. Start by taking 400 mg of magnesium a day. If your body tolerates that just fine, you can gradually increase the dosage to as much as 800 mg per day.

Though **manganese** doesn't play a starring role in fatigue prevention, it is a crucial member of the supporting cast. You body needs this mineral to process B vitamins and maintain steady blood-sugar levels...and all of that can keep your energy flowing. You can safely take up to 11 mg per day of manganese in its supplement form. Avoid taking this along with any of your other mineral supplements (especially iron and magnesium), though, as they will block each other's absorption.

Amino acids are called the building blocks of life. That's because they're the component parts that make up proteins, which are vital to every single organ system in our bodies. There are 21 amino acids needed for human life, some that your body can make on its own and some that it needs to get from the outside. (The ones you need to get from outside are called essential amino acids). When we don't eat right, we don't get the right mix or the right quantities of amino acids. And the primary symptom of an amino-acid deficiency is fatigue. You can get an amino-acid-complex supplement (that contains all of the essential amino acids) and take one pill two times each day. It's best to take these supplements on an empty stomach, so they don't interfere with the amino acids in your food.

> **The Doctor Is In**
>
> Your body's cells make its energy. When the enzymes needed for the process are in short supply, your energy will be too. One relatively new supplement, an enzyme called NADH, is showing lots of promise for patients with chronic fatigue syndrome—and it just may work for other kinds of ongoing fatigue.
>
> Adrenal Complex is another energy-boosting blend. This supplement contains a beneficial mix of ingredients that help stimulate your adrenal glands, reducing stress and increasing energy levels. You'll find fatigue busters like pantothenic acid (a B vitamin), Siberian ginseng, and licorice in this special blend. A word of caution, though: Folks taking anything that contains licorice root extract should make sure to get their blood pressure checked regularly.

You've probably been hearing a lot about how important **essential fatty acids** (like the ones found in fish oil) are to your overall health. Our bodies need these fats to run smoothly, and without big enough supplies you will end up feeling (you guessed it) fatigued. You can get your daily dose of EFAs in fish and fish oil and also in flaxseed oil. Just add one tablespoon of flaxseed oil into your favorite salad dressing at lunch time, and it will help get your energy levels back on track.

The Copper Connection

One common source of fatigue rarely talked about is copper imbalance. This trace mineral is essential for optimal health, but when you've got the wrong amount in your system, it can wipe you out. If you're tired of hearing that there's no medical cause for your fatigue, ask to have your copper levels tested—you and your doctor may be very surprised by the results.

Copper levels walk a very fine line between beneficial and detrimental. In proper amounts, it helps keep your body running smoothly. Check out some of its most important functions:

- Building collagen, which is needed for strong bones and connective tissues
- Forming hemoglobin and red blood cells by helping your body make the most of your iron supplies
- Decreasing free-radical damage to your tissues
- Regulating your thyroid function
- Keeping blood cholesterol at healthy levels
- Producing melanin, a pigment that gives color to your skin and hair

Since this mineral assists in so many crucial functions, imbalances can seriously disrupt your health...and it's very easy to unknowingly knock your copper levels out of whack.

The Zinc-Copper Competition

Zinc and copper form a precarious partnership in your body. The two compete for absorption, just like siblings do for attention, and only one of them can prevail. The problem with that is this: The two elements coexist in almost every cell of your body. In the right balance, they work together to keep you in peak condition. When they're out of balance, it throws off everything.

Copper imbalances can be brought on and made worse by zinc imbalances. Zinc can block copper absorption, so too much zinc cancels out copper. But when your body has too little zinc, copper levels can spiral out of control. The trick is to keep levels of both minerals in harmonious balance: 1 part copper to 8 parts zinc.

First, let's look at how much copper you actually need. The RDA is pretty low, just 900 micrograms, but you can safely take up to 10,000 micrograms a day if your levels are running low. When you don't get enough copper, that deficiency sets you up for things like rheumatoid arthritis, high cholesterol, iron-related anemia, fatigue, and weakness. On the flip side, too much copper can mess with the jobs of other essential nutrients, and that can cause overwhelming tiredness. Either way—whether you have too much copper or too little—one key symptom is fatigue. And, believe it or not, the imbalance usually leans toward copper overload.

Where the Copper Comes From

Copper is a very sneaky mineral, showing up in very unexpected spots. Surplus copper can squeeze out zinc, and that lets your body absorb even more copper. Here are some things that aid and abet copper as it strives to take over:

- stress: When you are stressed, your body loses zinc, giving excess copper a chance to take over.
- high blood sugar: Your body needs zinc to properly process sugar. High blood-sugar levels draw from your body's zinc stores, leaving the field free for copper.
- medications: Several drugs, including antacids and diuretics, impair zinc absorption, which paves the way for a copper coup.
- environment: Outside sources, like municipal water that uses copper sulfate for purification or household cleaners that contain xenoestrogens (which block your ability to eliminate excess copper), also add to copper imbalance.
- food: Low-fat/high-carb, vegetarian, macrobiotic, vegan—any of these diets can lead to copper overload, as they are unusually high in copper and low in zinc.

Chocolate Coins

Your overall diet plan can lead to a copper imbalance, but there are also particular foods that bump up the copper count all on their own. Chocolate, for example, has an extremely high copper count, making it among the worst dessert choices for people with copper overload. Other coppery food culprits include avocados, nuts, soy, dried fruits, shellfish, mushrooms, and tea.

Copper Tests

There are a few different ways to test copper levels. The most common are with blood or urine samples, and one of the best (but least used) is through tissue analysis. (Don't worry, they just snip some hair). Both blood and urine tests are capable of revealing extreme copper overloads, but they often miss the mark when the imbalance is less pronounced or on the deficiency side. Tissue tests, on the other hand, give a much clearer picture of copper levels.

Here's why: When your body senses a mineral overload, it treats the excess mineral as a toxin and works to move it out of the bloodstream into tissues... where it can be better dealt with. At the same time, copper only shows up in urinalysis when levels are enormously high. In addition, mineral levels in the blood and urine are immediate, based on what you ate, drank or breathed in that day. That gives your doctor a quick snapshot of your situation but hardly a long-term view.

Tissue mineral analysis can detect levels over a two- or three-month period, since tissues (including hair) act as mineral-storage facilities. Copper levels in your hair can be nearly 10 times what will be found in your blood, making the mineral much simpler to measure. The trouble with this method lies in its minimal use—a lot of labs don't perform the procedure properly, and a lot of sample analysts misinterpret the results. Plus, personal factors...like hair dye or perm solutions...may alter results, so be sure to wait for treated hair to grow out before collecting the sample.

The Potassium Problem

Another pair of minerals share a balance issue that's a lot like the copper-zinc one. Potassium and sodium, working together, supply power to every living cell in our bodies. Together, they play a key part in cell metabolism...when they're in the right balance. When they're out of balance—which is extremely common with a normal American diet—your body just can't function properly. And one of the biggest consequences of out-of-whack potassium and sodium levels is extreme fatigue.

Nature tries to make it easy for us to take in the right amounts of each mineral for our bodies. Potassium is plentiful in fruits and vegetables, so our bodies are built to run through it quickly because it's so easy to replenish. Sodium, on the other hand, is scarce in natural foods, so our bodies hang on to it for dear life.

What's even more important than how much of each we take in is the balance between them. As long as the ratio is right, it doesn't matter so much if we have a little or a lot of both. And there's the catch: Our normal diets are backward, and that messes with the precarious sodium-potassium balance. We eat tons of sodium (mainly in processed foods), and our bodies cling to it...but we get very little potassium (from fresh foods), and our bodies get rid of it quickly.

Bottom line: Most of us have too much sodium and too little potassium running through our systems. And potassium deficiency is known to cause chronic fatigue.

Restoring the Balance

It takes some doing to get your potassium and sodium intakes in good balance—you won't find the answer in the freezer cases or the packaged-food section of your grocery store. Processed foods—even minimally processed ones—have more sodium and less potassium than natural foods. To get the right balance, you'll have to fill your cart with things like fresh fruits, vegetables, nuts, and seeds.

Some of the best potassium sources include:

- pistachios (unsalted)
- sunflower seeds (unsalted)
- raisins
- watercress
- spinach
- beet greens
- avocado

- yams
- potatoes (with the skin)
- bananas

It takes a serving only about the size of your fist to get a healthy dose of potassium from these foods.

At the same time, try to avoid things that drain your body of potassium, at least whenever you can. Potassium depleters include things like caffeine, alcohol, diuretics, salt, sugar, and stress. Also, some antibiotics may block potassium absorption—ask your pharmacist about this whenever you start a new prescription.

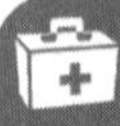

The Doctor Is In

Potassium is one of those minerals best gotten from whole foods rather than supplements. That's because getting too much potassium can cause as much trouble as getting too little. But if you just can't seem to get enough from foods, and supplementing seems to be the only choice, stick with potassium citrate supplements. They have been found to be well-tolerated and well-absorbed by most people, but don't take more than 500 mg at a time. Always take these supplements with food. And check with your doctor before adding potassium supplements to your regimen.

The Bounty of Sleep

It's tough to feel energetic when you're not getting enough sleep—in fact, it's tough to feel anything positive when you're exhausted.

Getting the Best out of Your Rest

Even when you are sleeping seven or eight hours each night, you may still wake up feeling tired and groggy instead of refreshed and energized. Those feelings of sluggishness could be due to poor sleep...and that can come from surprising problems in your bedroom. (No, not that kind of bedroom problem, environmental issues.)

First issue: allergens. Even if you don't think you have allergies, certain particles can cause uneasy breathing and disrupted sleep. In many cases, our bedrooms have extremely high levels of indoor contaminants—dust mites, pet dander, and formaldehyde (common in carpet padding), just to name a few. You can decrease these allergens by doing things like:

- using a vacuum with a HEPA filter
- washing your bedding at least once a week in hot water and drying it on the hottest dryer setting
- swapping your down pillows for the fiber-filled variety
- moving plants to other rooms
- getting rid of permanent-press sheets and switching to 100% cotton

You can also improve the quality of your sleep by moving some electronics away from your bed. EMFs (electromagnetic fields, produced by electronics) can affect your brain waves...and that could disrupt your sleep patterns. Try to keep electronic equipment at least 15 feet away from your bed. That includes the TV, your cordless phone, your clock radio, and lamps.

Chronic Insomnia

Insomnia hits all of us from time to time, but it's a constant problem for some folks. For some, it involves difficulty falling asleep. For others, the problem is staying asleep all night. And some poor folks get a double whammy, trouble falling asleep followed by a rude awakening in the middle of the night. Insomnia has lots of causes, and some of those are easily controlled, like caffeine intake or vigorous exercise late in the day. Some cases, though, are caused by underlying illnesses (like diabetes, hyperthyroidism, and arthritis) and won't go away until you can get those ailments under control. Plus, lots of prescription medications can interfere with your sleep cycle—you can check the package insert or on-line to

How High Is Your Sleep Debt?

Just like you can push the limit on your credit card, you can push yourself to the limit with too little sleep. That accumulated lack of sleep is called sleep debt, and it adds up over time. Here's how it works: If your body needs eight hours of sleep each night and you only give it six hours for two nights during the week, you've just built up a four-hour sleep debt. Credit-card debt costs you interest...and sleep debt costs you energy. Pay yourself back by getting enough sleep every night.

see if one of your medications could be causing this problem.

Sleeping pills are easy to get, and easy to take—but taking them is a bad habit to start, and a nearly impossible habit to break (not to mention that using them to deal with your sleep issue could be covering up a more serious underlying problem). Prescription drugs come with a long list of potential side effects and the risk of addiction.

Luckily, you can get all the benefits of sleeping pills in safer herbal preparations. Several very effective herbs can do the trick—giving you a good solid night's sleep without a morning-after hangover. Like **valerian**, a highly effective sleep aid proven to work in over 100 studies. This herb has been used for centuries to help insomniacs get to sleep. Take one teaspoon of liquid extract about 30 minutes before bedtime. (The maximum safe dosage is 2 teaspoons.) The next time insomnia strikes, try a different herbal remedy, like **kava**. European doctors frequently recommend kava for their patients who have trouble sleeping (as long they have no liver problems—see the sidebar for more on that). The best form of kava is standardized freeze-dried herb capsules. Start with 250 mg right at bedtime. (The maximum safe dosage is 500 mg.) You can also work milder herbs, like melissa (a.k.a. lemon balm) and chamomile, into your rotation. For these, simply steep the dried leaves in boiling water for about 10 minutes and drink one or two cups of the tea about 30 minutes before bedtime.

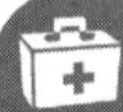

The Doctor Is In

Do not use kava more than two or three days each month—using it more than that could bring on some side effects. And do not use it at all if you have any type of liver disorder, since kava can make liver ailments much worse. Along those lines, do not take kava if you've had any alcohol or have taken any acetaminophen. If you do take any medications regularly, ask your doctor or pharmacist if they might impact liver function in any way (and let him know you're considering taking kava as a sleep aid). If his answer is yes, steer clear of kava while taking those medications.

In addition to using faster-acting sleep aids, you can try taking calcium and magnesium supplements on a regular basis as part of a possible long-term solution. Deficiencies in either of these minerals can cause insomnia, and getting sufficient supplies of them can correct sleep disorders.

The best way to use herbs to help you sleep is to find a few that work for you and use them in rotation. That way, your body won't build up a tolerance to any one herb. And remember, these herbs work much like prescription sleep aids—they make you drowsy very quickly—so don't take them unless you're ready to devote a good six hours to sleep.

Spend Energy to Make Energy

You know the old saying: "You have to spend money to make money." Well, the same is true for energy. Sitting around saps your energy, making you feel tired and sluggish. Moving around—even just a little bit—starts to get your blood flowing, moving oxygen and nutrients through your body.

Here are some things that a little bit of exercise can do for you:

Improve your cardiovascular system: Every time your heart beats, it sends blood throughout your body...and your blood pressure determines just how smooth that flow will be. Regular exercise evens out your blood pressure and strengthens your heart, so that every beat packs a bigger punch.

Strengthen your respiratory system: You need oxygen for energy, and breathing is the only way to get that. Exer

cise makes you breathe more deeply and rhythmically, giving your body its full oxygen requirements. This is especially true of aerobic exercise, which maximizes your oxygen intake.

Help you overcome depression: Exercise gets your neurotransmitters transmitting more actively, and that helps combat depression—a major cause of fatigue. In fact, working out specifically sparks production of serotonin and endorphins...some feel-good chemicals in your brain that have the great side effect of boosting your energy.

Help you sleep soundly: One key component of fatigue-fighting is getting enough sleep, and exercise has been proven to help people do just that. Get in a moderate workout at least four hours before bedtime, and you'll find sleep comes more easily.

Increase your stamina: Sure, you may be wiped out right after your workout, but over the long haul, your stamina will be greatly improved by regular aerobic exercise. In fact, after about four weeks of aerobic activity (three times a week for 30 minutes), you'll find that you're not even as tired during or right after the session anymore.

CHAPTER 7

A Razor-Sharp Mind

Millions of people worry about getting Alzheimer's disease or developing dementia, when the facts show that a relatively small percentage of people actually do. More likely, those annoying mental lapses are due to simple age-related forgetfulness—and that we can do something about. Though minor memory lapses are frustrating (Where are those #$%$ car keys?!), they don't signal impending brain disease or impairment. Even better, they are easy to prevent, and even possible to recover that instant recall you thought you'd lost. It's literally never too late to get your razor-sharp brain power back with a little bit of effort.

Your brain is greedy, the neediest organ in your body. To function smoothly, it needs a sufficient blood supply, a steady stream of high-quality nutrients, healthy nerve cells, and efficient neurotransmitters. All of those things diminish, at least slightly, as we age...and that can lead to memory and cognitive problems. Some of the most common causes of this loss include:

- atherosclerosis
- thyroid imbalances
- low blood-sugar levels
- shifting estrogen levels (especially in women)

- poor nutrition
- medications
- fatigue
- stress

You can combat all of those causes. You don't need expensive prescriptions, you won't have to follow complicated regimens. All you really need to do is add certain foods to your diet (or increase your intake), take a couple of supplements, go for a walk, and tease your brain. Hitting at least three of those four every day will get your brain in shape for mental gymnastics and instant-replay-like recall.

Think Food

Every organ in your body needs food, and some of those organs can get pretty picky about what they want—and none more than your brain. Your brain uses more nutrients and has more specific dietary requirements than any other part of your body...what you eat impacts how you think.

Lots of brain foods just happen to start with the letter B: berries, broccoli, beans, bread, Bordeaux. Plus, food rich in the B vitamins can do wonders for your gray matter. Add in some other letters of the alphabet, and you've got yourself a healthy-brain diet. By simply eating more of the foods discussed in this chapter, you can fight forgetfulness...defeat dementia...prevent Alzheimer's disease...and keep your brain running on full power.

Eat Your Breakfast (Burrito)

Your brain is hungry all the time, and after going a whole night without being fed, it needs some nutrients...pronto. That's why many studies have shown that skipping breakfast leads to lower test scores, lower productivity, and poorer performance overall. But you can't just fuel your brain with the regular stuff—especially first thing in the morning, when your brain needs premium fuel. A British study found the ideal breakfast includes beans and whole-grain toast, giving your brain plenty of protein, B vitamins, and fiber (which has also been shown to improve cognitive skills).

The best of the bunch may be berries, virtually all kinds. Turns out that berries have special antioxidant powers that appear to slow down—even reverse—degenerative brain diseases. Blueberries are at the top of the brain-health list. Animal studies in Mexico showed that a blueberry-rich diet could keep levels of a key protein in check, a protein called NF-kappaB that's connected to brain aging and memory loss.

Kidney beans also make the all-star list when it comes to brain support. This nutrition-packed food contains lots of thiamin (a.k.a. vitamin B1), which your body uses to make acetylcholine, a neurotransmitter responsible for memory. You'll also get a huge supply of iron, which creates the enzymes your neurotransmitters need to work properly. Folate, another crucial vitamin in kidney beans, also boosts neurotransmitter efficiency, which in turn boosts memory. And the heaviest hitter on this roster is tryptophan, a compound your body needs to make two extremely important neurotransmitters: serotonin and melatonin, both critical for optimal brain power.

Bread is probably already a big part of your daily diet—but when you switch to the whole-wheat variety, you'll have added a whole new dimension of brain protection. Whole wheat bread contains a lot of dietary fiber, and fiber's been proven to boost the energy supply to your brain. It's also packed with the B vitamins (especially thiamin) that keep your mind running. Plus, whole-wheat bread contains a healthy dose of Vitamin E, a known brain antioxidant that protects your fragile brain cells from oxidative stress.

Now add some broccoli to your menu. Broccoli contains compounds called lignans, and they've been shown to improve all kinds of cognitive skills. A British study conducted in 2005 showed that broccoli actually helps your brain in a second way—it keeps up production of a brain chemical called acetycholine, which is usually very low in Alzheimer's patients.

Round out your meals with a glass of wine. Thanks to a recent Japanese study, we now know that some wines contain special compounds (called peptides) that may delay or even prevent Alzheimer's disease. You'll find the highest concentrations of these brain-saving peptides in California Merlots, Sauvignon Blancs from

Bordeaux, and Pinot Noirs. On top of that, red grapes...and red wines...are rich in an antioxidant called anthocyanin (which protects your nerve cells) and reservatrol (which protects your brain cells).

Apples already enjoy a great reputation as healthy food, and now there's proof that they can reduce your risk of developing Alzheimer's disease. That's because apples contain lots of quercetin, a unique antioxidant that helps combat oxidative damage to your brain cells. In the lab, cells treated with quercetin showed substantially less DNA damage than cells treated with either Vitamin C or nothing. Those results add to the growing body of research that suggests that an apple a day can protect your brain.

Don't Forget the Fish

For generations, fish has been called "brain food." That's because it's one of the best sources of DHA, a nutrient your brain needs to flourish. Studies have indicated that taking DHA can improve concentration, even reverse memory loss. That's because this nutrient, along with other omega-3 essential fatty acids, helps your neurotransmitters keep things moving right along. These fats allow electrical signals to pass easily between your nerve cells, so messages that can get through. Plus, DHA, in particular, protects your cell membranes, which naturally break down over time.

Brain-Building Supplements

You can get a lot of brain fuel from the foods you eat, but some special supplements can take your thoughts even further. First up are those B vitamins, which your brain needs to keep in perfect working order. Next on the list is an amino acid called L-glutamine, one of the building blocks of brain power. Finally, we have a couple of herbs—Gingko biloba and gotu kola—that can do wonders for your recall and sharpen your thinking power.

To really boost your brain, load up on B vitamins—choline, folate, vitamin B6, and vitamin B12. People with higher levels of these B vitamins are able to hold on to their verbal and spatial-perception skills, according to a very large Veterans Affairs Normative Aging Study. Part of that is due to the homocysteine-fighting powers of B vitamins—because high homocysteine levels have been connected to poor cognitive function and recall skills. Choline plays a unique role in brain-boosting: Your brain uses it to keep its transportation system moving right along. Increasing your choline levels may help improve both the speed and the quality of your brain activity—like taking the express train instead of the local bus. Look for a B-complex supplement, one that contains the whole gamut of B vitamins and names specifically the four listed above. Make sure to take this supplement along with some food.

Another crucial brain nutrient is L-glutamine, one of the "nonessential" amino acids. Our bodies produce L-glutamine (that's what makes it nonessential), but production can drop off as we get older—especially when other stresses (like injuries or illnesses) get involved. The brain uses glutamine to create neurotransmitters and supply energy to the nervous system. Plus, glutamine protects your brain from ammonia poisoning—and you may be exposed to a lot more ammonia than you realize (in cleaning products, for example). High ammonia levels have been linked to neurodegenerative diseases, L-glutamine keeps those levels in check. To protect your brain from that danger, and to keep it in top-notch cognitive condition, you can safely take 1 gram twice a day, not with food (preferably on an empty stomach).

On the herbal front, Gingko biloba can work wonders for memory restoration. This herb has been tested heavily, with much success, but it does take some time for results to be noticeable—as long as three or four months, so you have to stick with it. Ginkgo works by improving the blood flow to your brain, a necessary component of optimal brain functioning. Take 350 mg of the freeze-dried whole herb (in capsule form) three times a day.

Gotu kola is a widely used herb that sometimes gets a bad rap because of its name. (It has nothing to do with cola.) But adding this supplement to your regimen can sharpen your

Performance Drugs

Feel like your brain is just moving too slow? There's a pill (or two) for that, with dozens more to come. "Cognitive-enhancement" drugs are already showing up on prescription pads around the world. The most popular—modanifil—started out as a treatment for narcolepsy, but researchers soon found out that it affected other people in a different way. Taking just one dose of the drug can keep you awake and alert for up to 90 hours (straight!) without the jitters or a scatterbrained effect.

mind...improve your memory...and even postpone age-related memory loss. Lab studies have shown that gotu kola helps animals learn and remember new behaviors more easily. And a human study found that the herb could improve concentration and attention span, even for developmentally challenged children. Take 400 to 500 mg of the crude herb (found in capsule form) three times a day.

Exercise Your Body to Enrich Your Mind

The results are in, and they're unanimous. To keep your brain in tiptop shape, you need to exercise your body. Dozens of studies have confirmed this, and most have found that more is better. That doesn't mean you have to exercise more strenuously, though, it just means you should spend more time being active than sedentary. In fact, a new U.S. study found that regular exercise can delay the onset of cognitive impairment—including dementia and Alzheimer's disease. And for this study, working out just three days a week was enough to make a substantial difference—up to a 40% lower risk of developing dementia.

Keep Your Brain Cells Dancing

As soon as you hit about 30 years old, your brain starts to lose tissue...and your mental agility goes right down with it. But you can slow that process down, even turn it around, with some aerobic exercise. A group of scientists did brain scans on 55 older adults—and the ones with the best cardiovascular health (thanks to regular aerobic workouts) had more brain tissue than their couch-potato counterparts.

You don't need a gym membership or fancy equipment. In fact, just walking—strolling even—for 30 minutes three times a week can boost your mental abilities by 15%. Walking more than that can increase your brain power even more. Plus, people who walk regularly show much less mental decline than their nonwalking peers. Here's why: Researchers from the Salk Institute found that physical exercise promotes new brain-cell growth...no matter how old you are!

Moving around increases your blood circulation—and that gets more glucose and oxygen to your brain, two key ingredients for mental agility. Exercise naturally increases your heart rate and breathing rate, which optimizes both energy production and waste removal.

You can start that process even before you get out of bed in the morning. As soon as you wake up, just move around—toe wiggling, stretching, rolling—anything that feels good. In fact, the simple act of wiggling your toes gets things going by waking up the nerves that stimulate your organs...including your brain. To keep that blood flow going, double back and retrace your steps from the bed to the kitchen before you settle in for breakfast.

> **The Power of Rest**
>
> Exercise is critical to a healthy brain, but its counterpart can't be overlooked. Sleep deprivation can literally wipe out your mental capacity. . . while a good night's rest can make all the difference to your focus, problem-solving skills, and memory. Fortunately, any brain function lost through lack of sleep can be easily replenished with 40 winks.
>
> And that's not all: Not only can sleep restore cognitive skills, it can also make them better. While you're asleep, your brain solves problems and processes new information. If you've been struggling to find the answer to something, give it a rest—that answer may just come to you in your sleep.

Brain Training

You know the phrase "Use it or lose it," and that truly applies to your brain. The best way to protect your brain cells is to work them, the harder the better. In fact, your brain gets its biggest benefits from struggling, from trying to figure something out or learn something new—the bigger the challenge, the bigger the bump in brain activity. When you work your brain, you build new neural connections and strengthen the ones that are already there. And that's what will keep your cognitive skills and memory intact.

> **Bingo!**
>
> Believe it or not, bingo is good for your brain. First, it gives you a social connection that boosts your cognitive reserve. Second, it gives your hand-eye coordination a robust workout. Third, it puts your short-term memory into overdrive—you've gotta know what's on your card if you want to win.

For you folks who like to see the numbers, here's a pretty impressive one: Brain exercises can reduce your risk of developing Alzheimer's by up to 64%! The more you do, the more your risk drops. That's what a group of Chicago researchers found when they studied 6,158 people (all at least 65 years old). The folks who scored the highest on the cognitive-activity scale—and they scored higher when they exercised their brains more—had the lowest incidence of Alzheimer's. And we're not talking about algebra problems or complicated puzzles here...the activities included things like reading the newspaper.

> ### *The Brain Bank*
>
> There's mounting evidence that what protects you from losing brain power is something called cognitive reserve. That's a lot like a mental-storage facility, and the better-stocked it is, the longer it takes to run out of brain power. What gets put into the reserve? Everything you learn and do. In fact, strong evidence suggests that a life full of stimulating leisure activities—brain games, socializing, travel, and the like—builds up the brain-power reserve enough to hold off mental decline.

Mind Your Music

If you've got grandkids, you may have heard about the Mozart effect—a theory that says listening to classical music stimulates brain activity. Various studies have been done to try to prove that one way or another, and the jury is still out on whether listening to music actually boosts brain function. Playing music, on the other hand, is another animal entirely—and many studies on this have shown that children who can learn to play music score better on spatial-reasoning tests.

Music lessons do involve a lot of key components of brain training. Like using both hands to work both sides of the brain...like focusing on rhythm and pitch... like precision hand movements. Now, no studies have been done to measure the mental impact of playing music on older folks, but it certainly makes sense to try it.

Mind Control

There's a new New Age-type brain exercise in town, and it's slowly but surely gaining some scientific credibility. It's called neurofeedback, and it works by letting you actively control your brain activity.

Neurofeedback grew out of its sister science, biofeedback—a way to control particular body functions by your will (functions like body temperature and heart rate). Though many patients learned how to do this successfully, they couldn't really explain how. Now the science of listening to your body's messages and making changes based on those messages can be applied to your brain function too.

The first stabs at seeing how well this worked involved brain-wave activity measured by an EEG machine. Researchers tried to have patients increase the size of their alpha waves, which are largest when we're relaxed and focused. They did this with a sort of video game, where bigger alpha waves could make a car go faster—and it worked. That success led to more experimentation, and now neurofeedback is being used to treated some brain-related ailments: epilepsy, anxiety, and strokes, just to name a few.

Brain Aerobics

To keep your brain in tiptop shape, you have to work it harder. In fact, brain training is a booming business over in Japan, where about 20% of the population is age 65 or older...and that percentage is expected to increase to 25% over the next 10 years. From special sections in bookstores to weekly courses with names like "Healthy Brain Class," the Japanese take brain exercise very seriously.

Turns out that a 10-minute brain workout every day can do wonders for your memory, and even improve the mind function of dementia patients. And all you have to do is solve some math problems, crack some word puzzles, or even play specially designed video games. Some of these brain-training video games were met with skepticism by their new audience—until people began to see the results, that is. Many game users saw almost immediate results in

The Old Switcheroo

One great way to strengthen and build neural connections is to switch hands when you're doing simple tasks. Give your dominant hand a rest and use the other one to brush your teeth, eat, clip coupons, even change the channels with your remote. Sounds simple, but it's actually hard when you first get started. In fact, it may feel extremely awkward and uncomfortable...but that will pass. As your "weak" hand gets stronger and tasks become easier, ramp up the difficulty level—write your grocery list with your off hand, crochet "backward," or switch your tennis racket to the other side.

improved recall and thinking skills.

Double Up

Focusing on two senses at once can get your neurotransmitters working at double speed. All you have to do is split your focus when you're doing something you always do. Try to concentrate on the way your food looks as well as how it tastes. Or you can try to do two completely different sensory things at once, like listening to music while you squish Play-Doh with your grandson. Looking for more two-timing ideas? Try these, and remember to focus on both activities at once:

- Smell some flowers while you look at a painting.
- Pet your dog while you listen to a book on tape.
- Sniff a brain-boosting essential oil (like grapefruit or peppermint) while you knead dough.
- Look at pictures of someone you love while talking to him or her on the phone.

Pressure Swings Mess With Your Mind

A new study found that big variations in your blood pressure during the day can cause cognitive problems like forgetfulness, wandering attention, trouble finding the right words, and even disorientation. Dips and spikes in blood pressure can be caused by lots of things, including short-acting blood-pressure medications. You can help keep your blood pressure on a steadier course by keeping your potassium and sodium levels in good balance and by increasing your calcium intake. You can safely take up to 500 mg of calcium twice a day, best taken along with magnesium.

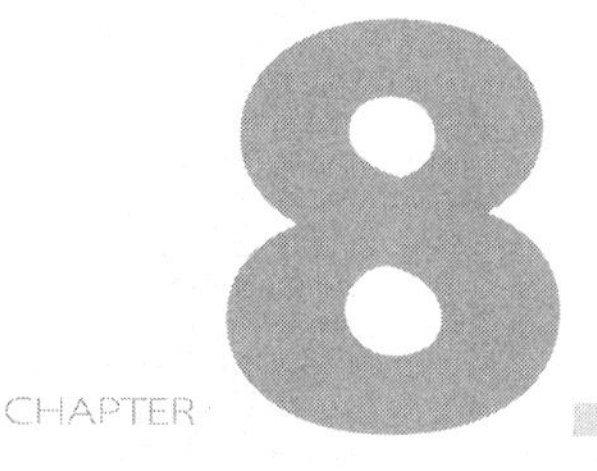

Defeat Depression and Diminish Stress

Depression affects about 21 million Americans every year. Stress (I'd guess) affects about 21 million Americans every day. Both of them weigh on your physical and mental health, and both can cause irreparable damage if not treated. Not only that, but each can make the other worse, and they both tend to be long-term issues.

Though the effects of these conditions can be very different, they do have a lot in common. In many cases, treating one helps treat the other—and many natural healing methods can work to ease either condition. Conventional medicine, on the other hand, often treats only the most obvious symptoms, ignoring underlying causes. The quickest fixes often seem to be pills—antidepressants, antianxiety drugs, sleeping pills. And in the case of severe stress, the symptom treatments are more likely to be things like high-blood-pressure medications, cholesterol-lowering medications, and the like. While these medications may be called for in some cases, they may also complicate the situation with side effects that add to the stress and depression.

What Exactly Is Depression?

People throw the term "depression" around like a softball, but it's a lot more than just feeling down. It's the medical term for a physical/emotional condition that comes with a long list of possible symptoms, including:

- persistent sadness, anxiety, or emotional emptiness
- feelings of hopelessness, helplessness, or guilt
- loss of interest in the things you usually enjoy (anything from gardening to reading to sex)
- low energy, fatigue, and just feeling slower
- indecisiveness, memory problems, confusion, and lack of focus
- insomnia or excess sleeping
- unusual weight gain or loss
- thinking about death and suicide

Keep in mind that most people will have some of these symptoms at one time or another, even the most severe ones. The main distinction that makes me diagnose true depression is that the symptoms last for a long time—days, weeks, or months, rather than popping up just once in a while for a day or two. Depression may cause only one of the symptoms listed above, or it could bring on quite a few of them. If you have even one of these symptoms and it has lasted for more than a day or two, consider getting some help.

Depression can be brought on by an event (like the loss of a loved one or losing your home), an illness (like stroke, cancer, or Parkinsons' disease), hormonal shifts, genetic predisposition, and stressful situations. In fact, lots of times it's a combination of factors that sets off a depressive disorder.

Stress: the Good and the Bad

Nature gave our bodies a great tool to use when things get out of hand: stress. When something bad was happening to our ancestors (like being chased by a pack of wolves), their stress feelings provided an efficient emergency-management system, pumping up all of the necessary hormones to get them out of that frying pan and into a safety zone. It happened fast, they got out of trouble, it was over, their bodies relaxed. That's the good part of stress.

Now, however, many of us live under near-constant stress. And that continual state of emergency keeps our hormones out of whack and keeps our bodies in a virtually never-ending state of panic. Increased heart rate, shallower breathing, muscle tension...these reactions are great when trouble shows up. In our lives, though, the trouble never leaves, we never get to the safety zone, and we never fully relax. That wreaks havoc on our bodies, causing some damage to critical systems (like cardiovascular, endocrine, and nervous).

A Bit of Biology

When stress shows up, your adrenal glands go into overdrive and produce lots of cortisol (the stress hormone). Constant stress can keep those adrenal glands out of balance all the time, pushing cortisol production to dangerous levels. To cut back on cortisol production, you need to restore balance in your adrenal gland...and you can accomplish that by boosting your DHEA (another hormone, with a very long tongue-twisting name) levels. DHEA supplements are widely available. And if you're more comfortable with a gentler approach, you can take some daily Siberian ginseng—which contains a compound your body needs to create its own DHEA.

Who's Really the Happiest?

Here's a puzzler for you: Most people believe that unhappiness grows as we get older, but the truth is quite the opposite. Several studies show that, contrary to popular belief, most people get happier every year. There are a few theories about why that may be so, like the fact that most of us are more settled in our lives when we're older than when we were younger...or that we're better able to adapt to changes because we've already lived through so many of them...or maybe because our lives begin to focus more on our own enjoyment and personal relationships than on achievement and work.

One study involved two groups, 273 people with an average age of 31 and 269 people with an average age of 68. All of the subjects were asked a bunch of questions about their own happiness (past, present, and expected future) and also about how happy they thought 30-year-olds and 70-year-olds were in general. Almost all of the subjects assumed that happiness generally declines as people get older—the complete opposite of the individual results, where the older people reported being happier than the younger people did.

Make Connections

According to my cousin Rose (who got it from Barbra Streisand), people who need people are the luckiest people in the world. Whether you like the song or not, there's a lot of science backing it up. People with family, friends, or even pets fare better than folks who go it alone.

You may feel like you have no control over connecting with other people, but you do. You can start attending religious services. You can volunteer, go to the senior center, join a reading group, or sign up for an exercise class. Not every connection you make will turn into a lifelong friend, but you've got to start somewhere.

I know it's not always easy to get yourself out and about—if it were easy for you, you'd probably be doing it already. So start small: You can talk to the produce guy at the grocery store...ask the librarian to recommend some books...or strike up a conversation with a neighbor. The more you talk to people, the easier it will get, and the better you'll feel.

This is especially true for women. One study in particular found that one of the best ways a woman can avoid depression is to build a strong support network. Feeling cared for, and being smack in the middle of a positive social circle acts like an innoculation against depression. The study included around 1,000 sets of opposite-sex twins, each pair raised in a single home (so this is not one of those eerie separated-at-birth studies). This way, they shared genes and a common environment but not gender. All participants were interviewed twice (with at least one year between sessions) and screened for depression. And the women with higher levels of social support had the lowest incidence of depression, though the social support-depression connection was not as strong for the men. (Just an aside, the only kind of social interaction that *didn't* cut the risk of depression for women was interaction with their own children.)

In case you're feeling left out, guys, the Australian Longitudinal Study of Aging points to men with tight social circles living longer than their antisocial counterparts. For 10 years, researchers followed 1,477 men and women, all over age 70. They found that people with big networks of friends lived longer than people whose circles consisted only of family ties, no matter how strong those were.

Hug Power

Ever feel like you just need a hug? That could be because hugging is a double-edged version of the healing touch (like you'd get from a massage). Numerous studies have shown that touching and being touched cause measurable, positive physical changes in both people. That gives a simple hug the power to ease anxiety and depression, and just plain make you feel better.

Relax and Rejuvenate

Most of us live in pressure cookers, dealing with all sorts of demands from dozens of sources, demands our ancestors never even dreamed of. Every day we face the frustration of commuting, the pressure of taking care of our families, demanding jobs, constant communication (cell phones, E-mail, instant messaging, pagers—it's almost impossible to escape). For all the conveniences of our world, we pay a huge price...and that price often comes at the expense of our mental and physical health. No surprise there, as the two are securely intertwined. In fact, stress and stress-related complaints are the leading reasons for trips to the doctor—some surveys say up to 90% of all visits!

Both our mental and physical well-being are affected by outside factors, some under our control and some not. When problems come up, lots of doctors reach for prescription pads...and sometimes that may be the best course. More often than not, though, finding ways to relax and reduce stress levels works better and faster (and without any nasty side effects).

There are several different relaxation and stress-reduction techniques out there, all safe and effective, but the ones I've seen the most success with include:

- meditation

- deep breathing
- yoga
- acupuncture

You may need to try out a few different approaches until you find the one that relaxes you and makes you feel refreshed. Whichever technique you decide to go with, do it for at least 20 minutes every day, as sort of a daily relaxation break. You can also turn to your method of choice in times of extreme stress to help take the edge off—like doing some deep breathing when your grandson has been crying for the last three hours and your daughter won't be back for another hour...or performing a mini-mediation when your boss decides to redefine the project you've been working on for the past two weeks and wants the changes by Friday.

Meditation

Everyone has his own favorite meditation technique. Mine involves serene surroundings and a focus phrase. (Mine happens to be "beer and pretzels," but you can choose any word or phrase that's important to you.) Add to that a comfortable position and a passive attitude, and you have all the ingredients for a successfully relaxing mediation.

Here's how it works:

1. Get yourself into a quiet spot away from ALL distractions (no cell phone, no pets) and sit in your most comfortable position.
2. Close your eyes and become aware of your breathing.
3. Relax each of your muscles, starting at your forehead and working your way down to your toes...and imagine your tension blowing away with each exhale.
4. Breathe at your normal relaxed pace, silently saying your focus phrase every time you breathe out.

Keep this going for 10 to 20 minutes every day. To keep yourself from constantly glancing at your watch, set a timer for your chosen meditation period. When the timer goes off, continue to sit quietly for a few minutes, sort of like a cool-down period after exercise.

Deep Breathing

Changing the way you breathe can literally change your life. Controlled deep breathing can dramatically improve how you feel by increasing the oxygen flow throughout your body. Breathing more deeply and less frequently accomplishes just that. Think about it: Anxious breathing...characterized by quick, shallow breaths...often leads to hyperventilation and a serious lack of oxygen, making you feel even more anxious. Doing the opposite has the opposite effect—a calming one.

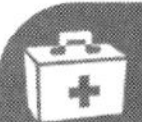

The Doctor Is In

Don't worry that you aren't doing this right—there is no one right way to meditate. And worrying about your meditation defeats the purpose! Try to keep your mind as relaxed as your body. If any stray thoughts wander in, shoo them out by refocusing on your focus phrase and your breathing.

Try this tension-taming deep-breathing exercise. And don't be surprised if you find yourself actually relaxing!

1. Stand with your feet slightly apart and your arms hanging relaxed at your sides.
2. Breathe in through your nostrils, causing your lower abdomen to puff out. As you inhale, imagine the oxygen flowing throughout your body.
3. Breathe out (loudly) through your mouth, letting your abdomen deflate. As you exhale, imagine that your tension and anxiety are flowing out of your body. (Expect to feel your muscles unclench as you release this tension.)
4. Repeat until you feel relaxed.

Yoga

Yoga provides kind of a mixed bag of relaxation techniques. It combines some physical exercise with controlled breathing and meditation, all three of which are known to combat stress. Regular yoga sessions come with another triple benefit:

- improved blood circulation
- enhanced muscle tone and flexibility
- increased levels of feel-good brain chemicals

That trio of benefits work together to defeat depression and soothe stress. And it gets better: Yoga has the added bonus of being a weight-bearing exercise, which promotes strong bones.

There are many different kinds of yoga, all with slightly different angles but with the common themes of breathing, specific poses, and meditation. The one you'll hear the most about in the United States is hatha-yoga (which happens to be the kind I practice).

The best way to learn yoga is to take classes with a qualified instructor. Sure, there are tons of do-it-at-home videos, but it's easy to tie yourself into pretzels if you haven't had some human guidance first. (Take it from me: Get some lessons before you try this at home!)

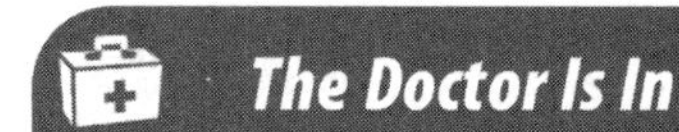

Choose your acupuncturist carefully. Most states require these traditional-medicine practitioners to be licensed—and that license is based on specific skills and education qualifications. You can check with the National Certification Commission for Acupuncture and Oriental Medicine (at www.nccaom.org) for a list of certified practitioners in your area.

Acupuncture

Acupuncture and its no-needle cousin, acupressure, have been used in traditional Chinese medicine for thousands of years. By now, practitioners have the techniques down pat, and millions of people rely on acupuncture to keep their *qi* (life force) flowing in balance. Practitioners believe that *qi* imbalance or blockage is the root cause of all disorders, and that includes overstress, depression and, anxiety.

In acupuncture, tiny needles (really tiny, about the width of a hair) are inserted into particular points on your body. There, they stimulate your *qi* to get it flowing right. (With acupressure, these same points are stimulated with pressure instead of with needles.) Along with restoring qi flow, acupuncture and acupressure help your body restore its natural balance...and produce feelings of vitality and well-being.

Natural Ways to Soothe Your Mind

Life is hard—and nature knows it, providing lots of ways for us to keep depression and undue stress in check. These natural methods are often gentler on our systems than prescription drugs but just as powerful when it comes to making us feel better.

Nothing is going to turn depression around overnight, and no one can just "snap out of it." Natural treatments may take a little longer to kick in fully than prescription drugs, but they're far less likely to cause unpleasant (or dangerous) side effects...and that makes it a lot easier to stick with them. What can you expect if you turn to one (or more) of these natural remedies? To feel a little bit better every day, until suddenly you realize that you feel fine.

Bring on the Sun

Depression can be brought on (or made worse) by a lack of good ol' sunshine. One ailment in particular, seasonal affective disorder (or SAD), is directly caused by diminishing natural light...but its effects can be reversed with a healthy dose of sunshine or some time in front of a light box.

Try to get outside for at least an hour a day (it doesn't have to be all at once) during peak sun hours. You don't have to sunbathe to get the benefit; just expose your eyes to some sunshine. (Of course, don't look directly into the sun!) Sun exposure can jump-start your adrenal glands and help keep those stress hormones in better balance.

Movement and Mood

There's more and more evidence that exercise can boost your mood, but this is definitely not a quick-fix solution. A long-term commitment to working out regularly—even lightly—can bring about a long-term change in your mental well-being.

One of the most recent studies in this area (now called neurobiology) found out how exercise affects neurological processes. Your central nervous system controls things like your mood and stress level—and physical activity can alter the messages it sends out. Researchers plan to learn just how this works, and exactly which messages can be adapted. For now, it looks like stress messages can be toned down and happy hormone messages can be stepped up.

Another study, this one about the long-term effects of aerobic exercise in folks over 60, found that working out brought on real improvements in some psychiatric symptoms. The longer people participated, the bigger the change—and the people who stuck with it the longest (14 months) demonstrated the most improvement.

For those of you who prefer gentler workouts, you'll be glad to hear that yoga can improve your overall well-being and quality of life. A recent study of 135 Americans (ages 65 to 85) found that practicing yoga qualitatively improved quality-of-life scores on some standard scientific scales.

Feel-Good Supplements

Some people will tell you that depression and anxiety are all in your head—they're only partly wrong. Those conditions can be caused by brain-chemical deficiencies, a situation that can easily be remedied with some supplements.

SAMe

S-adenosylmethionine (a.k.a. SAMe, pronounced Sammy) is my supplement of choice for treating general depression naturally. In the first place, your body produces SAMe all on its own—it's just that production slows down as we get older. One of its key jobs is breaking down brain chemicals so our bodies can use them, chemicals like serotonin (the good-mood chemical). Without enough SAMe, we can't break down enough crucial chemicals, and that can lead to depression. When you supplement with SAMe, you're back in the feel-good game.

There's plenty of research to back this up. SAMe has been proven more effective than placebo in clinical trials, at least when it comes to treating depression. Even better, studies have shown it to be just as effective as antidepressant drugs but without any of their common side effects (headaches, insomnia, loss of libido, and impotence). And even better than all that, it seems to work faster than drugs, which can take up to eight weeks to kick in, while SAMe can bring you back in just half the time.

Start by taking 800 mg of SAMe daily, split into two doses. If your stomach can handle that with no problem, work your way up to 1,600 mg per day (also split into two doses). If you do get an upset stomach, drop the starting dose back down to 600 mg per day (split into two doses) and work your way up from there.

GABA

Gamma-aminobutyric acid, or GABA, is one of the amino acids produced by your brain. It's also one of the key neurotransmitters that help minimize stress-related impulses. Usually, your brain creates enough GABA to keep you on an even keel. But sometimes outside factors can mess with that balance...things like a poor diet, or too much exposure to environmental toxins (like pesticides). When that happens and you're GABA-deficient, feelings of anxiety, irritability, and depression can take hold.

You can supplement with GABA, and it can make you feel much calmer. In fact, it works like Valium and Xanax but without the overwhelming threat of addiction. You'll find GABA along with other amino-acid supplements at your pharmacy. To combat stress, take 250 mg three times a day, away from food (at least one hour

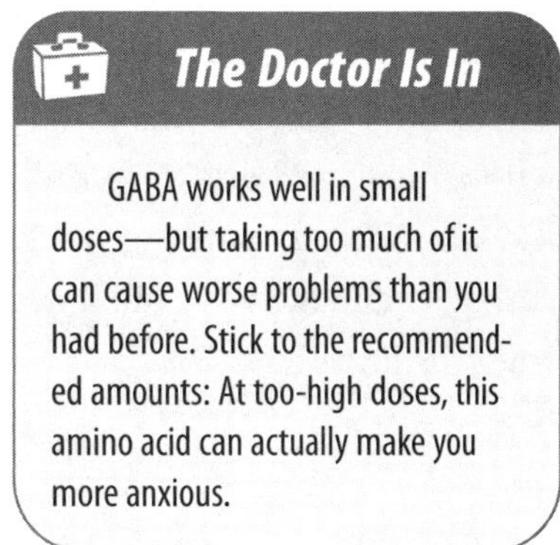

The Doctor Is In

GABA works well in small doses—but taking too much of it can cause worse problems than you had before. Stick to the recommended amounts: At too-high doses, this amino acid can actually make you more anxious.

before or two hours after you eat). If you're already taking a prescription drug for anxiety, talk to your doctor before you take any GABA.

L-Tryptophan

Tryptophan is an amino acid, one that your body uses every day in dozens of ways. One of its most critical roles is as an ingredient—your body can't make serotonin (the feel-good hormone) without it. When production of tryptophan is low, you may start feeling low, so replenishing this essential nutrient is a great first move. And in case you're worried about having too much, don't—you literally can't take too much of this stuff.

The supplement form of this amino acid is L-tryptophan, and it's readily available in capsule form. Just 500 mg per day—which, conveniently, is the only dosage it comes in—will do the trick to ease anxiety and depression. Here's the trick: Never take this supplement with any other protein. (They compete with each other, so your capsule will be wasted.) Also, don't take it with a meal, and don't use milk to wash it down. Wait a couple of hours after eating, then take your pill with some water or juice.

Tryptophan Gets a Bad Rap

The story starts back in the 1980s, when medical doctors throughout the United States began recommending L-tryptophan supplements for their depressed and suicidal patients. This natural solution proved effective and protective—as pills couldn't be hoarded and used in suicide attempts like traditional sleeping pills. Its success was so evident that the CDC estimated that as many as 14 million Americans were taking the supplement.

The big twist came in 1989, when a Japanese manufacturer skimped on quality and produced some L-tryptophan supplements that caused a deadly disease called EMS. Even though experts were able to trace the problem directly to the Japanese manufacturer—in fact, directly to a specific production lot number—the FDA banned all L-tryptophan from public sale. The ban began on March 22, 1990. And, perhaps coincidentally, just four days later, *Newsweek* put out a cover story about Prozac, a "breakthrough drug for depression."

Twist number two—a much lesser known twist—came in February 1993, when the U.S. government issued a patent for the use of L-tryptophan to treat EMS. . . the very disease that brought on the U.S. ban!

The Other Side of Antidepressants

Antidepressants are among the most commonly prescribed drugs in America, but not the most commonly taken. In fact, a 2003 study uncovered a surprising statistic: 65% of patients surveyed reported they'd stopped taking their medication...and half of them said it was because of the side effects.

That doesn't surprise me, though. A lot of the side effects of commercial antidepressants are similar to the symptoms you're trying to get rid of! The newest generations of these drugs (like Prozac, Paxil, and Wellbutrin) do have fewer side effects than earlier forms (like Elavil and Tofranil), but they still come with a long list of things to look out for. Some of the more common side effects include:

- excessive sleepiness
- insomnia
- increased anxiet
- unusual weight gain or loss
- disappearing libido
- suicidal thoughts

Any of those sound familiar? (They should, they're all common symptoms of depression.) Add to those things like nausea, vomiting, diarrhea, headaches, and dizziness, and it's easy to see why people just stop taking them.

Here's the big "however:" Despite potential problems with the drugs, they do help millions of people conquer depression when used in conjunction with other methods (like talk therapy and relaxation techniques). If you're taking antidepressants and they are working for you, don't stop until your doctor says it's time. In fact, if you're taking antidepressants and they're **not** working for you, don't stop taking them without talking to your doctor.

Electricity Can Brighten Your Day

It's not shock treatment—not at all like scenes from *One Flew Over the Cuckoo's Nest.* Today's electronic stimulation mirrors your brains own natural electrical impulses. After all, that's what your brain does; it sends impulses through the neurotransmitters to let you know what you're feeling. With a little bit of electrical intervention, your depression can be lifted.

Back in the '90s, the Liss Cranial Stimulator (LCS) was beginning to gain recognition in psychological fields. This pioneering tool could increase or decrease the activity levels of particular neurotransmitters, changing the effect they had on mood. Studies showed that the LCS method of administering high-frequency electrical impulses had some measurable effects, like higher levels of:

- serotonin, the feel-good hormone
- endorphins, which can make you feel ecstatic
- GABA, the body's "natural tranquilizer"
- DHEA, a hormone that may play a key role in depression

Along with those good increases came declines in cortisol (the stress hormone) and tryptophan (which can make you sleepy) levels. That combination of changes had a very positive impact on depression.

As Far as the Eye Can See

Many people just expect to lose their sight as they age. They may not expect to lose it completely, but just try to imagine someone "older" without picturing reading glasses. Millions of people mistakenly believe that vision loss is inevitable, a normal part of the aging process. While it's true that our sight distance may dip a bit, and that reading glasses may indeed become part of our wardrobes, serious vision loss is not something to accept without a fight.

The biggest cause of severe vision impairment and blindness in the United States isn't aging—it's age-related diseases that strike the blow. That's a big difference, because even though there are a lot of sight robbers out there, many can be treated and some can be easily prevented. Statistics say that by 2040, there will be twice as many Americans affected by disease-related vision loss as there are now. I say, let's try to avoid that club.

That's not to say your vision won't change as you get older. It probably will. Many people can't read the fine print as well as they did when they were younger. Some people see "floaters," tiny spots that float across their field of vision, especially in very bright light. Still others may have dry eyes, which can make your eyes itchy and uncomfortable—or the opposite, wet eyes, when your tear ducts go into overdrive and your eyes are filled with tears. These are extremely common conditions and usually aren't anything more than annoying. Sometimes, though, they can be signs of bigger problems to come, which you can prevent if you catch them in these early stages. As soon as you experience a new symptom, no matter how small it seems, see an eye specialist.

The Top Four Sight-Stealing Diseases

1. macular degeneration
2. glaucoma
3. cataracts
4. diabetes

Here's the good news: These diseases are preventable. And if you're already dealing with one or more of them, a lot of treatments are available...and more are being developed every day. Whenever the prevention path is still open, I tell people to jump on it—it's easier to protect your eyesight than recover it.

Macular Degeneration

AMD (or age-related macular degeneration) slowly destroys clear central vision. It can hit one eye or both, and this disease can make it impossible for you to enjoy everyday pleasures like driving, reading, and watching TV.

AMD comes in two forms: dry (much more common) and wet (much more dangerous). About 90% of people with AMD have the dry variety, and doctors still aren't sure what causes this. And even though only about 10% of people with AMD have the wet kind, it causes 90% of the blindness. This form works much faster to steal your central vision.

Trouble is, you won't get much warning. Neither form of AMD causes pain, and vision loss is usually so slow that you won't notice it until it's really gone. It will just get a little harder to see all the time—harder to see the freckles on your grandson's nose, harder to read the paper. Slowly but surely, you'll develop a blind spot right where your central vision used to be. People with wet AMD may have one more obvious symptom: Straight lines may start to look crooked.

On the plus side, there's a lot you can do to prevent AMD from ever destroying your vision—even substantially slow the progress of the dry version of the disease. For example, the AREDS (age-related eye diseases study, a huge clinical trial) found that taking a particular combination of antioxidants and zinc could help preserve vision. That combo includes a daily dose of 500 mg of vitamin C, 400 IU of vitamin E, 25,000 IU of vitamin A (a.k.a. 15 mg betacarotene), 80 mg of zinc oxide, and 2 mg of cubric oxide (copper). You'll also find several other natural ways to protect your eyes from AMD throughout this chapter.

Glaucoma

Did you ever get that annoying eye-puff test at the eye doctor's office? Well, that's one of the key tests for glaucoma. In combination with the dilated-eye test (also not the most pleasurable experience), your eye doctor may be able to catch glaucoma before it steals your eyesight.

Glaucoma works by increasing the

The Amsler Grid

As part of your eye exams now, expect to see the Amsler grid (a common diagnostic tool for detecting AMD). It's basically just a checkerboard with a dot in the middle. If you have early stage AMD, the straight lines of the grid may look distorted when you look at it with one eye covered at a time.

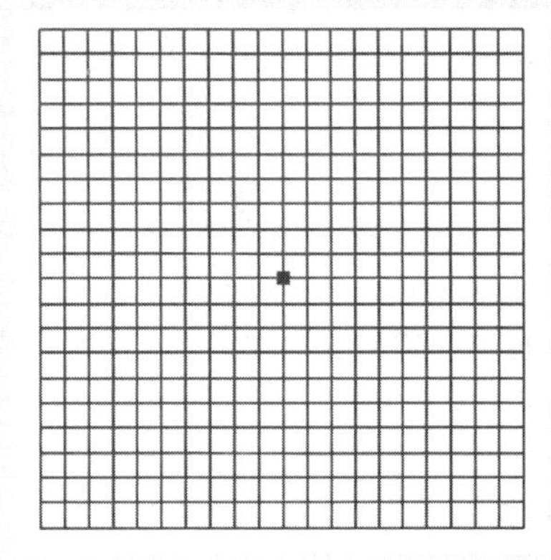

An Amsler grid, as seen by a person with normal vision.

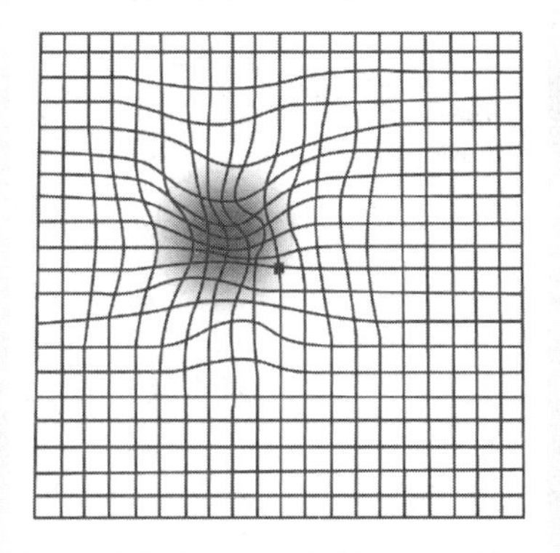

An Amsler grid, as it might be viewed by a person with age related macular degeneration.

(Images courtesy of National Eye Institute, nei.nih.gov)

fluid pressure in your eyes until that pressure starts to do some damage. As the pressure builds up, it gets harder to see out of the corner of your eye. And as the disease progresses, your field of vision will get narrower and narrower until all you have left is central vision...or no sight at all.

The bad news is that there's no known cure...but there are things you can do to prevent or control glaucoma before it causes full-blown blindness. Prevention is the meat of this chapter, and the following sections talk about all the different things you can do to keep your eyes in tiptop shape. On the control front—which comes after you've been diagnosed and before your eyesight is gone—there are traditional eye drops and pills you can use. These medications work in one of two ways to keep your eye pressure down: Some slow down the flow of fluid into your eyes, and some boost fluid drainage out of your eyes. Either way, less fluid means less pressure and a better chance of preserving your eyesight. On the down side, these medications come with some side effects and, worse, often stop working over time. And on the simple side, avoiding dietary stimulants like caffeine can help lessen the tendency toward increased pressure.

Cataracts

I've heard lots of patients refer to cataracts as "cloudy eye," and the nickname fits. The condition is caused by clumpy proteins in your eye that band together

The Real Cost of Lucentis

In June 2006, the FDA approved Lucentis, an injectable eye treatment for folks with the wet version of age-related macular degeneration. Lucentis got that stamp of approval because of a study in which it appeared to maintain vision for more than 90% of patients who got monthly treatments for a year. That's what makes the headlines...here's what doesn't: About 60% of the patients who didn't get Lucentis also maintained their initial level of vision at the 12-month mark. Commonly reported side effects included eye pain, bleeding eyes, increased eye pressure, and inflammation. In some cases, Lucentis treatment also caused retinal detachment and traumatic cataracts. And if you can get past all that...and can deal with getting injections *in your eye,* be prepared to cash in some bonds: A single treatment can cost anywhere from $600 to $2,000, and it takes at least three to see any improvement.

and blur your vision, just like a small cloud blocking your focus. As time passes, that cloud—the cataract—can get bigger, making it even harder to see. And while two of the biggest risk factors for cataracts are smoking and diabetes, anyone can get this disease. In fact, you may have tiny cataracts in your eye right now that are too small to even notice.

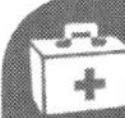

The Doctor Is In

Think twice before you opt for eye surgery to handle glaucoma... and then think again. Laser surgery has shown some success when it comes to eye-fluid drainage. But the effect wears off over time, and you'll probably have to keep taking drugs anyway. Regular surgery also works by widening the drainage pipe, but it poses some big risks (like causing blindness) and is usually used as a last resort.

The only way to truly detect cataracts is with an eye exam. So if you think your vision is getting cloudier, make an appointment. The gold-standard treatment for cataracts is surgery, and it has a pretty high success rate. It's actually one of the most commonly performed operations in the United States, topping 1.5 million procedures every year. But—and this is a big but—just because you may have some cataracts doesn't mean you should get prepped for surgery. Most cases aren't severe enough to warrant that treatment.

The big news here is prevention studies. The National Eye Institute (part of the NIH) is looking into natural prevention methods, like vitamins and minerals, that just might stop cataracts right in their tracks (as you'll learn later in this chapter). Researchers are finally catching up with what I've been talking about for years—let's just hope their clinical trials come up with the kinds of results naturalists have seen for generations.

Diabetic Eye Disease

As you can guess from the name, diabetic eye disease is brought on by diabetes—particularly when blood sugar isn't kept under tight control. The name actually refers to a group of conditions that the disease can cause, including diabetic retinopathy (the most common). Diabetes can also increase your risk of developing glaucoma and cataracts. But you can cut down your risk of developing diabetic retinopathy and other vision-stealing conditions by staying on top of your glucose levels.

Diabetic retinopathy is the number one cause of blindness in adult Americans—sad, because it is easily preventable through disease management. Basically, it causes changes in the blood vessels in your retina, and those changes can cause severe vision loss and even complete blindness. But, and here's the tricky part, this disease comes with no obvious warning signs. In fact, there are often no noticeable symptoms in the early stages. It doesn't hurt or cause vision changes until fairly late in the game.

What you can do to catch this as early as possible is to get regular eyes exams. If you have diabetes, get at least one exam each year, and be sure it includes getting your eyes dilated. When a qualified eye professional catches the early stages of retinopathy, he can treat it with laser surgery. "Early stages" is the key phrase here—the surgery can be used to prevent vision loss, but it can not restore vision already lost.

Wide Open

I can't say this enough: Get your eyes checked at least once a year and be sure your pupils get dilated. It's the ONLY way to catch some of the worst eye diseases, the ones you won't notice until it's too late to get your sight back. No one likes having this test done (including me), but do it anyway. Bring double sunglasses and a designated driver, and just get it done.

The Sight-Protection Diet

Bugs Bunny had it (mostly) right all along: Some of the best defenders of your vision are as easy to find as a bag of carrots at the grocery store. More and more research is confirming the link between specific foods, especially fruits and vegetables—and eyesight. So where did Bugs get it wrong? Turns out that fruit provides even more protection than vegetables, though vegetables are a very close second.

One major study—really major, with a whopping 118,428 participants—found that you can lower your risk of developing macular degeneration by 36% simply by eating at least three servings of fruit every day. Another study (this one included over 50,000 women ages 45 to 67) found that getting a lot of Vitamin A from foods decreased the risk of getting cataracts...by up to 39%! And people who eat cantaloupe (according to yet another study on this subject) can cut their risk of needing cataract surgery right in half.

Now, you probably already know that cantaloupe is great for your eyes (thanks to plenty of vitamins A and C). Here are some more foods that pack a mighty protective punch for your eyes:

- Dark, leafy greens: From kale to spinach to collard greens, these veggies all contain generous amounts of betacarotene (which converts to vitamin A). On top of that, dark-colored greens also contain lutein and zeaxanthin (two antioxidant compounds proven to protect your eyes against macular degeneration).
- Cherries and berries: These tiny fruits contain huge amounts of flavonoids, powerful compounds that safeguard your sight. When you're picking them, remember—the darker, the better.
- Red wine: One glass of red wine provides a flavonoid cocktail, with quercetin, resveratrol, and rutin, all of which combat oxidative stress that can lead to retina damage. And a study of 3,072 adults found that drinking moderate amounts of red wine regularly could protect against macular degeneration, by preventing it in the first place and by slowing progression if it has already started. Plus, rutin has been shown to reduce eye pressure—and that can help you avoid developing glaucoma.
- Fish: Australian scientists found that people who eat a lot of fish rich in omega-3 fatty acids are much less likely to develop macular degeneration. Their study included almost 2,900 participants with an average age of about 64. The ones who reported eating fish at least once weekly were 40% less likely to end up with the disease. Fish on that eye-protection list include salmon, mackerel, herring, tuna, and sardines.

Supplement Solutions

When it comes to eyesight, it takes three kinds of supplements to fully arm your arsenal: vitamins, minerals, and herbs. Sometimes, you can get sufficient vitamins and minerals from foods. Other times, you've just got to take the pills to get enough dosage to make a difference. As for the herbs, capsules are really the best way to get the standardized blend and the right amounts.

Vitamin A is critical for optimal eye health and is particularly effective in combating glaucoma. In fact, vitamin A deficiency has been directly linked to the condition. You can get a lot of this nutrient from foods high in betacarotene but probably not enough to treat your eye troubles. For that, you'll need to supplement with 10,000 IU of vitamin A daily. That's not all, though: In order for that vitamin A to be used by your eyes, it needs a zinc chaser—so take it along with 15 mg of zinc.

Vitamin C is found in high amounts in lots of fresh foods—but you still need more to make a real difference here. On top of that, vitamin C can leave your body as quickly as it got in, so it needs to be constantly replenished. Several studies have linked increased vitamin C intake and the resulting rise in blood levels with a substantially decreased risk of developing cataracts and glaucoma...but you have to take a lot of it. Start with 500 mg three times a day. That may sound like a lot, but it's nowhere near the maximum safe level. In fact, you can safely take up to 1,000 mg per hour every day; your body will let you know when it's had enough (by increased urination and loose stools). If your body gives the signal, cut back on your dosage.

Lutein and zeaxanthin are carotenoid antioxidants, and large amounts of both can be found in your eyes—especially on your retinas and lenses. Though few clinical trials have been conducted to learn more about the connection between high levels of lutein and lowered risk of sight-stealing diseases, there's plenty of trend

Smokin' Herbs

Since the early 1970s, we've known that smoking marijuana can lower eye pressure (called intraocular pressure, or IOP), a critical part of defeating glaucoma. Scientific studies have confirmed that it really works in every form—smoked, through an IV, eaten (in a pill)—except topically to get that IOP down. Due to its reputation as a recreational drug, research tailed off when more conventional treatments came on the scene...so no one really knows just how well marijuana stacks up against other treatments. The only thing we do know for sure—it works...but it's illegal to use it without a prescription.

evidence (meaning people who get a lot of it through food and supplements fare better) out there proving its worth. Some research has shown that these antioxidants can protect you against macular degeneration and cataracts...but, again, you need to consume quite a bit for the true protective effect. One successful study had people taking 10 mg of lutein daily, about double the normally recommended dosage—that level was safe and effective, and showed clear restoration results.

B Vitamins, particularly vitamin B12 and folate, offer strong protection against cataracts. This was proven conclusively in the large Blue Mountains Eye Study of 2001, in which researchers found a direct connection between folate and B12 supplements and substantially lower risk of developing cataracts. Try 1,000 mcg of B12 along with 400 mcg of folate. These vitamins work best when taken together in sublingual form.

Selenium helps your body produce a substance called gluthathione, which protects your eyes from ultraviolet light—a major cause of damage. In fact, you can't produce any gluthathione, which is vital to cataract prevention, without sufficient stores of selenium. This trace mineral works best when taken along with vitamin E, which has also been shown to offer protection against cataracts. The two nutrients combined are more effective than either is on its own. Look for a supplement that contains 400 mcg of selenium and 400 IU of vitamin E and take it once a day.

Fish Oil contains plenty of omega-3 fatty acids and makes a great substitute for people who just don't like eating fish. Just pop a capsule or two every day with food, and you'll get plenty of protection. Overall, take 1,000 mg per day.

Ginkgo biloba appears to stop retinal problems right in their tracks and offers special protection against macular degeneration. In clinical trials, Ginkgo has been proven effective for correcting vision problems caused by this debilitating condition. It may also fight glaucoma, as this herb is known to improve blood flow. The best formulation is one standardized to 24%. (It will say that right on the bottle.) Take 120 mg, twice a day.

Bilberry extract, at least according to the stories, helped British pilots hit their targets during World War II. It seems that when they ate bilberry preserves before a bombing, their night vision would be sharper. Whether those stories are true or not, the results of clinical trials are—and they say that the high levels of flavonoids in bilberry extract appear to stop vision loss and sharpen existing vision. Look for an extract that's standardized to 25% (just check the label) and take 240 mg twice a day.

Exercise Your Eyes

Even folks without any of the major eye diseases can see their vision deteriorate a little bit over time. That's why we see so many people wearing reading glasses or bifocals. But there is a way to regain some of your lost vision...without medication, without laser surgery, and without risky side effects. All it takes is a little bit of time every day, thanks to an amazing eyesight-restoration program created by W.H. Bates.

With just a few simple exercises, you can relax and strengthen your eyes and improve your vision. Even if you've worn glasses for a very long time, you may be able to get rid of them when you follow the Bates program. Try some of these easy eye workouts...and see your vision get better.

Palming

Bates discovered that we can all have perfect center vision when we focus properly—it's just that we don't usually do that. To get that 'central fixation' (as he calls it), you need to stare at a blank surface—which you can do with his palming exercise. Warm up your hands, close your eyes, and then gently cover your eyes with the palms of your hands so that all the light is blocked out. (Don't put pressure on the surface of your eyeball while you do this.) If you "see" total blackness behind your eyes, continue resting just like that for five minutes. Do this exercise three or four times a day.

The Other Kind of Exercise

Full-body exercise helps your whole body stay healthy. . .including your eyes. One of the biggest benefits of a good workout is improved circulation. That brings more vital nutrients to every part of your body, head to toe. And since many eye ailments are brought on by nutrition deficiencies, improving circulation can help make sure that nutrients make it to your eyes.

If you don't see pure black, don't worry—lots of people see kaleidoscope colors at first. Here's how to get to the black: Imagine a small black dot while still palming. Then let that dot grow bigger and bigger until it fills up the whole space behind your eyes.

Eye of the Needle

Acupuncture may help protect your vision—and, no, you won't have to get needles in your eyes. Turns out there's a strong connection between low blood flow to your head and macular degeneration... and acupuncture can restore normal blood pressure. That neat little trick can improve your vision, near and far, by 69%!

Shifting, Swinging, and Flashing

No, this isn't a new exotic dance—it's a set of Bates eye exercises. The first, shifting, started with a standard Snellen chart (you know, that eye chart in your doctor's office where they make you try to read lines and lines of shrinking letters). Bates found that this chart could be used to improve vision...and not just make you feel like you can't see. His advice: Get a Snellen chart, hang it up in your house, and then do this shifting exercise every day: First, look at any letter on the chart; then shift to another letter that's a few spaces away but on the same line. After that, shift back and forth between those two letters five times. Next, look at a large letter near the top and then shift down to one of the smaller letters near the bottom. Shift back and forth between those two letters five times.

Swinging involves more of your body. Stand with your feet about a foot apart, facing one wall of the room. Pick up your left heel and turn your eyes, head, and shoulders to the right until your shoulders are parallel with the wall on your right. Then do the same motion in reverse: Lift your right heel, and turn your eyes, head, and shoulders toward the left-side wall until your shoulders are parallel to it. Do this exercise three times a day, with 30 full-swing repetitions each time, to start. Work your way up to 100 complete swings in each set.

Flashing brings us back to the Snellen chart. For this exercise, you get to rest a little. First, rest your eyes for a few minutes; then palm your eyes for a few minutes (using the palming method described above). Open your eyes for just a fraction of a second and look at a letter on the Snellen chart. Then close your eyes and rest them. Repeat this opening and closing exercise 15 to 25 times every day.

CHAPTER 10 Hear, Here!

Do you ever have trouble understanding what people are saying to you? Whether you're on the phone with your grandkids or in the doctor's office for your checkup, missing part of the conversation can come back to haunt you. Maybe you just promised to send Sonny $50 to buy a new video game...or inadvertently told your doctor you take a multivitamin every day when you don't. If you didn't catch the whole conversation—and were too embarrassed to ask for a repeat—you could be missing out on some critical information (like whether Sonny accepts checks, or cash only).

A lot of people associate getting older with hearing loss, mainly because most of us lose at least some hearing ability as we age. The numbers are deafening: Nearly a third of all Americans ages 65 to 74 have hearing problems...and about half of the people over age 74 suffer from hearing loss. Regardless of whether that loss is considered small or large, it's a big problem when it's happening to you. And if you just ignore it, it will probably get worse.

Here's the good news: There's a lot you can do to prevent or stall hearing loss, even some things you can do to recover (at least some of) your lost hearing. The first step is to figure out exactly what's going on. That determination will lead you to the best treatment, and the best chance of once again hearing a pin drop.

Plain Ol' Presbycusis

Age-related hearing loss—or presbycusis, as they call it in the medical books—isn't just about getting older. Sure, it's more common in older folks and tends to come on slowly and get worse over time. But aging is not necessarily the cause...and that gives us lots of room to turn things around and turn up the volume. Here are some of the many causes of "age-related" hearing loss:

- aging (had to put that one in here)
- long-term exposure to loud noise
- heredity
- circulation problems (including high blood pressure)
- medications
- illnesses and infections
- head injuries
- clogged ears

In addition to having many possible causes, presbycusis comes with a few different effects. The degree of hearing loss varies widely from person to person. And it may vary even in your own ears, with one losing more hearing than the other.

Are You Losing Your Hearing?

Hearing loss often creeps up on you, and often goes unrecognized in the early stages. But when the problem is detected early, treatment can do the most good. If you're experiencing at least one of the effects below, it may be time to start preserving your hearing:

- ❑ you have trouble hearing voices on the phone
- ❑ you have difficulty understanding high-pitched voices (like women and children)
- ❑ you can't follow the conversation when more than one person is talking
- ❑ people complain when the tv is at a good volume for you
- ❑ you can't separate primary noise from background noise
- ❑ certain sounds suddenly seem extremely annoying or especially loud
- ❑ you think everyone around you is mumbling

Along with the list of causes comes a long list of potential solutions. Mainstream doctors tend to go right for quick solutions—hearing aids, cochlear implants, and the like—rather than trying to reverse the problem and restore hearing naturally. In some cases, those steps may be appropriate. Much of the time, though, natural methods (like the ones you're going to read about in just a moment) will go a long way toward getting your hearing back.

Care for Your System, Care for Your Hearing

A lot of hearing is based on tiny impulses, how they're triggered within your ears and how they're received by your brain. If there's even one glitch along the way, your hearing becomes impaired—and aging can cause some definite glitches. As we get older, some of those impulses don't travel quite so quickly anymore, and sometimes part of a message gets lost in translation. That can happen as hair cells die, as neurons (nerve cells in your brain) lose their function, and as synapses (travel gateways for message transfer) lose their connectivity. But you can strenghten this whole message-sending system with particular nutrients that support its key functions.

Choline, a B vitamin, is a crucial component of acetylcholine, a brain chemical responsible for the quick transfer of signals. When levels are low, message sending slows down. But by increasing your choline intake, you can shore up your acetylcholine supplies and get things moving at top speed once again. The best way to accomplish this is by taking lecithin supplements, since they contain a choline source that doesn't break down until it gets to your brain. Consider taking 600 mg of lecithin two times a day to keep those connections sharp.

Vitamin E appears to protect your inner ear from the ravages of aging. Studies have shown this potent antioxidant can prevent damage to the ear's sensory hairs—even when they face direct attackers (like certain anticancer drugs known to induce hearing loss). Free-radical damage is believed to be a major cause of hearing loss. Vitamin E is a well-known free-radical neutralizer. Getting plenty of vitamin E can help scavenge those free radicals before they irreparably damage your hearing. Look for it in the form of 'mixed tocopherols' whenever possible—or at least as the d-alpha form, instead of dl-alpha. You can safely take up to 1,000 mg of vitamin E every day.

Coenzyme Q10 (a.k.a. CoQ10) shows a lot of promise when it comes to preserving precious hearing. At least one study found that this antioxidant could delay the progression of hearing loss in some subjects, particularly those with a family history of the condition on the mother's side. Treatment with 75 mg of CoQ10 twice a day was enough to halt the development of hearing loss that was already in progress.

Treating the Underlying Cause

Ears are delicate. Lots of common illnesses and infections affect them, as anyone who has had a very bad cold might know. Often, minor systemic infections will clog up your hearing temporarily—when your head clears up, your ears will be fine. Sometimes antibiotics may be called for, as in the case of bacterial infections; again, when the infection is gone, normal hearing is typically restored.

Some conditions that may affect your hearing aren't mecessarily temporary, conditions like high blood pressure and diabetes. Still, getting good control of those kinds of conditions can make the impact on your hearing a temporary one. Both high blood pressure (directly) and diabetes (indirectly) can mess with your circulation and blood flow when levels aren't kept in check.

And then there's Meniere's disease, a condition that may affect your ears in different ways: You may experience hearing loss, tinnitus, or stuffiness in at least one ear. The direct cause seems to be a change in fluid volume inside the ear...but no one knows what causes that. What we do know is that about 5 million Americans suffer from Meniere's disease and suffer from some form of hearing impairment because of it. Here's the tricky part: This condition is hard to diagnose, so it often gets missed. The hallmark symptoms—in addition to hearing problems—include vertigo, dizziness, nausea, and vomiting (usually because of the vertigo). If you've got this combination of symptoms, ask your doctor about Meniere's disease. That leads me to the topic of proper treatment (though, sadly, there's no cure) for this chronic condition. Lots of doctors jump on the drug bandwagon here, prescribing some combination of anti-vertigo medicines, anti-nausea medicines, and diuretics. I prefer the lifestyle-change approach, which has shown great success. The lifestyle changes that seem to get all the symptoms under control include cutting back on caffeine, salt, alcohol, and nicotine. (Yep, this is another push to quit smoking.)

Deafening Drugs

There are several medications out there that can damage your ear to the point of hearing loss. The solution: Stop taking them! (Talk to your doctor first before ever discontinuing a prescribed medication.) Some of the more commonly taken, well-known hearing robbers include:

- antibiotics: erythromycin, vancomycin, tetracycline, streptomycin, tobramycin, amikacin, and gentamicin (Note: These are the generic names, and some have multiple brand names.)
- antimalaria drugs
- chemotherapy drugs: Platinol, Ancobon, and Blenoxane (Note: These are the brand names.)
- aspirin

Again, don't stop taking these medications without talking to your doctor first. But if you've noticed hearing loss that suspiciously coincides with your medication's start-date, talk to your doctor about that. He may be able to switch your protocol before any permanent hearing loss sets in.

Ear Candling

Sounds a little crazy, ear candling, but it really works! Here's what happens: A special clothlike candle is placed in your ear and set afire. That creates a sort of vacuum between your ear canal and the candle, which draws out all sorts of gook (mainly wax build-up and excess fluid). For people with very waxy ears or a tendency toward ear infections, ear candling can help keep that canal clear. A clogged canal can cause muffled hearing; clearing it out can restore sharp hearing.

You can find ear candles at many health-food stores. They're much bigger than you'd probably imagine, the size of 10-inch tapers rather than birthday candles.

Another possible surprise: The candles are hollow and sort of conical, rather than dense like wax candles are.

Though the directions on the package say you can use them on your own, it's really much easier to work with a partner. Here's what to do:

1. Mark the candle about 2 inches above the bottom.
2. Cut a small circle in a paper plate, large enough for the candle to fit through snugly, and then put one candle through that hole until the plate is on that 2-inch mark.
3. Lie on your side and place the bottom of the candle (opposite the wick end) gently into your ear, with the plate falling slightly above your car.
4. As your partner (or you) steadies the candle and plate with one hand, she lights the candle with the other.
5. The ear candle will begin to burn down, and you will hear crackling and popping sounds, and may feel a slight sucking sensation in your ear.
6. Watch the candle. When it has burned down to about one inch above the plate (which takes about 25 minutes), your partner will remove the candle from your ear and then blow it out.
7. Cut open the candle and see the gunk that's been clogging up your ear. (Yes, there's a precise medical term for it—but that really just translates to a fancy way of saying "gunk.")

Repeat the process with the other ear. You can use ear candles about every other week to keep those canals clear.

Noise-Induced Hearing Loss

One of the many causes of hearing loss is noise, hence the diagnosis called noise-induced hearing loss (or NIHL). More than 10 million Americans suffer from this condition—but permanent damage can be preventable, and new damage may be reversible. If you are constantly exposed to noise, or have been forced to endure even one extremely loud noise, the best time to start protecting your hearing is right now! The sooner you start, the better you'll hear.

Natural Protection

According to research, antioxidants are among the most promising hearing protectors. That's no big surprise, as these nutrients seem to be able to do just about anything. Not only can some antixoidants help prevent hearing loss, but some have been shown to reduce existing NIHL (meaning you could regain some lost hearing!). One animal study showed that a diet full of vitamins A, C, and E, along with selenium, diminished NIHL—and that means increasing hearing capabilities. Then there's magnesium, believed to have a protective effect, possibly due to its ability to increase blood flow. A couple of Israeli studies found that taking 167 mg of magnesium could minimize the damage of hazardous noise exposure, limiting the amount of permanent hearing loss.

> **In Your Ear**
>
> Without launching a full-fledged biology lesson, here's what you need to know about how your ears hear: Hair. That's right. Your inner ear is home to tiny, delicate hairs that conduct the nerve impulses that your brain recognizes as sounds. Excessive noise, constant noise exposure, and super-loud sounds do damage to those hairs. That damage causes hearing loss, which gets worse over time.

In addition to those familiar nutrients, promising clinical trials have been conducted using some less familiar supplements. Such as NAC (n-acetylcysteine), an antioxidant that protects tiny hair cells and knocks out loitering free radicals. To protect your hearing, try taking 1,000 mg of NAC daily. It's best to take your NAC in two doses, each time away from food (at least one hour before or two hours after eating). And because NAC supplementation can alter the amount of zinc that passes out through urine, be sure you're getting some supplemental zinc as well.

Living With Tinnitus

Tinnitus remains a medical mystery—one that affects about 50 million

Americans. This condition makes you hear sounds that aren't really there...ringing, hissing, buzzing, roaring, whistling. The sounds can be high-pitched or low, constant or sporadic. Tinnitus can come on suddenly or gradually and can impact one or both ears. No one knows exactly what causes it, and there's no one right way to treat it. But there is one thing we do know: Suffering from tinnitus does not mean you're going to lose your hearing.

Even though there's no one definitive cause for tinnitus, it does seem to occur along with particular conditions:

- anxiety
- depression
- high blood pressure
- Meniere's disease
- food allergies
- diabetes
- thyroid imbalance
- Lyme disease

In most cases, treating the underlying condition will at least ease the symptoms of tinnitus, and sometimes will get rid of it altogether.

Sometimes, though, nothing makes the ringing (or buzzing or hissing) go away, and it starts to interfere with everyday life. For those folks, there are still things that can help make tinnitus easeir to deal with, even if they can't get rid of it completely. One of the biggest issues pertaining to this condition is the sheer annoyance factor, and letting it stress you out can make the symptoms worse (which causes more stress, which makes the symptoms even worse...you get the picture). Finding your best coping mechanism is crucial to managing tinnitus, and not letting it get the better of you.

The Mainstream Response

If you head to a conventional doctor and mention a constant buzzing in your ear, chances are he'll write you a prescription for antidepressants. Since many cases of tinnitus are linked to depression and anxiety (though it's not always clear which condition is the cause and which is the effect), that's the standard go-to treatment. Some of these medications have helped some patients better deal with tinnitus, but there's no conclusive proof that they're not just masking some other problem. On top of that, virtually all chemical antidepressants come with a whole host of unpleasant side effects...especially when you aren't truly depressed in the first place.

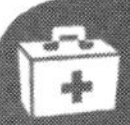

The Doctor Is In

Beware Xanax! Xanax (a.k.a. alprazolam) is an antianxiety medication normally used to treat people who suffer intense panic attacks and is often prescribed for tinnitus. Trouble is, it's highly addictive, so it's not appropriate for long-term use. Sure, it works (at least for the short-term) for some folks—one study found that 76% of participants experienced a 40% reduction in tinnitus symptoms. But part of those results may be due to the fact that Xanax just plain knocks some people out. Plus, the recommended course is a mere four months of treatment (to avoid addiction problems), and then you're on your own again.

And speaking of masking, another very common treatment does just that: mask the problem. Sometimes this is done through the addition of an external sound to sort of cover up or refocus your hearing, making the buzzing (or hissing or whooshing) less prominent. That typically comes in the form of a hearing-aid-like device that generates a constant noise. The problem with this: Lots of folks get equally annoyed with the masking sound, bringing them back to where they started.

What Really Works

Fortunately, there are several ways to manage your tinnitus—all safe and natural. Some of these methods may work well for you, others may have no effect at all. Because of the many possible causes of the condition, different treatments will work in different circumstances. Don't get discouraged if you try something and nothing happens...just keep trying until you find the treatment that works for you.

Start with relaxation, which comes close to being a magic bullet when it comes to dealing with tinnitus. For almost every sufferer, relaxation techiniques make the condition easier to deal with...and for some, it may get rid of the problem altogether. Stress and tinnitus often show up together, each making the other worse. By controlling your stress reactions, you can at least minimize the impact of the noise and possibly erase it. There are several proven relaxation methods out there, like meditation and guided imagery. Choose whichever one you like best, and let yourself begin to relax.

Nutrition also seems to play a role in tinnitus treatment, though you probably won't hear that from your doctor. Several essential minerals have shown promise for tinnitus patients—the trick seems to be getting the supplemental dose down pat. One of them (zinc) comes with clinical-trial data to back it up; the rest are based on anecdotal evidence, but appear to be quite successful. Even with the proper dosage, though, expect this treatment to take some time. It can take up to six months to see a substantial improvement in your symptoms, but stick with it, because if this works for you, it's a long-term solution. Here are the minerals and the dosages that have worked best:

- zinc, 90 to 150 mg per day (and be sure to balance it out with copper supplementation to avoid an imbalance between these two competing minerals)
- calcium, 1,000 mg per day (best split into two doses)
- magnesium, 160 mg per day
- selenium, 70 mcg per day
- manganese, 9 mg per day

In addition to minerals, B vitamins appear to play a key role in controlling tinnitus. Vitamin B deficiencies have been linked to the condition, and daily supplementing with a B-complex appears to solve the problem in many cases. When this treatment does the trick, results are generally seen within four months. Be sure the supplement you take contains at least 100 mg of thiamin (vitamin B1), 50 mg of vitamin B12, and 50 mg of niacin (vitamin B3) along with the rest of the B bunch.

A couple of herbs may also alleviate tinnitus symptoms. Ginkgo biloba appears to effectively improve tinnitus symptoms. Studies indicate that a daily dose between 120 mg and 240 mg may alleviate tinnitus. Start with the lower dose and continue with that for six weeks. If you don't feel, or rather hear, a noticeable improvement, bump up your dosage to the high end of the scale. You should begin to see the change in about four weeks. Another herbal extract, vinpocetine, has also shown success in silencing tinnitus. This herb seems to boost blood flow, thereby increasing your brain's supply of oxygen and glucose. That, in turn, improves tinnitus symptoms. And in one study, taking 40 mg daily improved those symptoms by 66%.

Sound Sleep

Insomnia may also cause tinnitus, or make it worse. Luckily, there's a solution with a one-two punch, knocking out both conditions with one tiny little pill. Melatonin, sometimes called the sleep hormone, is normally produced by our bodies. When production is off, our sleep cycles get out of whack...and for some folks, that's sets off a bout of tinnitus. Taking just 3 mg of melatonin every night appears to improve sleep and diminish tinnitus symptoms, according to the latest study—making it a great choice to turn off that ringing and get you sleeping soundly.

Hearing the Future

There's a lot of research going on about hearing loss right now, mainly connected with genetics and hair-cell regrowth. Much of this research is still in the infancy stage, and meaningful treatments may take some time to materialize...but they are out there, and innovative solutions could show up sooner than we expect. Here's a look at what's going on in labs around the world:

The Genetic Connection

Belgian scientists uncovered a direct genetic connection to hearing loss in older adults—flaws in just one little gene appear to trigger hearing loss even in the absence of no other risk factors. This mutation, dubbed KCNQ4, may play a key role in age-related hearing loss. And now that we know what to look for, we may be able to predict much earlier who is predisposed to hearing troubles and begin preventive measures before permanent damage is done.

Return of the Hair Cells

The most common cause of age-related hearing loss is the death of hair cells in the ear. We all start out with about 50,000 of these tiny hairs, and start losing them as we age. Unlike most cells in the body, these don't regenerate—once they're gone, they're gone. Or so we thought. U.S. researchers just discovered that turning off a particular gene leads to a lot of new hair-cell growth, at least in mice. Lots more research needs to be conducted before we'll know whether this works in humans and is safe. (No one really knows what will happen if we start turning genes on and off at will.) What the current research brings is hope—hope that merely restoring hair cells will restore hearing, hopefully without causing unintended damage elsewhere in the body.

Vitamin E Conquers the Unknown

Some people lose hearing suddenly—and in about 85% of those cases, no one can figure out the cause. Of that bunch, almost two-thirds spontaneously recover hearing in just a few days. . . but the rest don't. One group of researchers tried Vitamin E supplements on people hospitalized with idiopathic sensorineural hearing loss (a.k.a. sudden hearing loss with no known cause). Guess what? It worked, at least most of the time. Just 400 mg of the powerful antioxidant, taken twice a day, boosted hearing recovery—75% showed improvement by the time they left the hospital, and even more did at a later follow-up.

CHAPTER 11

Separating Truth From Fiction

People over age 50 are big business these days. There are more of us than ever before, and corporate America plans to sell us everything they possibly can. At the same time, scientific advances are coming at a fast and furious pace—but today's miracle/wonder drug/cure/anti-ager could be tomorrow's "pulled off the shelves" story.

This combination of science and slick marketing is irresistible. After all, who's not looking for that magic elixir to stay young, vibrant, and healthy? The trick is in sorting out the snake oil from the real deal...and that can be very hard to do.

The latest research focuses on a few key areas that scientists suspect could extend human life:

- human growth hormone
- calorie restriction
- dental health
- longevity genes
- lengthening telomeres

The jury is still out on whether any of these avenues will actually pave the way to a longer healthy life...and what potential dangers exist.

HGH and the Hormone Gang

Human growth hormone (a.k.a HGH) is being held out by some as the cure for aging—"Take this stuff, and you'll feel younger, longer." Lots of folks do swear by this, lining themselves up for HGH prescriptions from willing doctors. Can it really do the trick?

Let's back up a minute and talk about HGH. This is a hormone your body produces naturally while you're—you guessed it—growing. When you get to your physical potential, production slacks off because it's time for you to stop growing. Then some people found out that treating fully grown people with HGH appeared to stave off, possibly even reverse, some of the common complaints of aging. But through the roar of the crowd's enthusiasm, I hear a lot of questions and doubt.

Here are my three primary objections: First, you can get monthly HGH injections...for an exorbitant fee, now hovering about $1,500 per treatment! Second, there's the "why not?" factor: "If it might work, why not try it?" This concerns me because of a biochemical mechanism called feedback inhibition. That's where your body, in its ultimate wisdom, decides to take the easy way out—when it gets HGH from the outside, it can slack off and stop natural creation of the hormone. That's not a huge problem in the short-term. But as your body makes less and less of this hormone over time, it won't be able to pick up the slack if you suddenly decide to quit getting the injections. Third, there's a complete lack of long-term experience. We have no idea what the potential long-term consequences are, because HGH simply hasn't been used by fully grown adults before.

Luckily, there is an alternative: You can grow your own. The results may take a little bit longer, but the method is much more appealing. You can encourage your body to make more HGH on its own simply by supplying more of the raw materials that lead to its natural production. That way, your body is doing the job and you're not messing around with a perfectly effective system by injecting foreign hormones.

All you have to do is supply the raw materials, which are readily available, and they can stimulate your body's own growth-hormone formation. Arginine and ornithine are two amino acids that can spur production, and one is all you need. Arginine is the more commonly used, but either one will do...as long as you take it properly. To be effective, arginine (or ornithine) must be taken in 1,000 mg doses. Don't take it with food, or it will have to compete with other proteins for space on your body's protein receptors, which will dilute the it to the point of uselessness.

Here's the caveat: Have your hormone levels monitored by a nutritionally oriented doctor, starting with a baseline reading (meaning *before* you start any kind of treatment, even supplements). Then, get regular follow-up lab tests to make sure your levels are where they should be. You and your doctor can modify treatment as needed.

Extremely Low-Calorie Diets

One of the latest antiaging discoveries is the calorie connection. It seems that eating an extremely low-calorie but high-nutrient diet slows down the natural aging process. Some research supports this plan...but, frankly, I can't get behind it (the plan, not the research). Sure, it may work. It may even work so well that you can add five or 10 or even 20 years on to your lifespan. As for me, I don't want to spend even five or 10 or 20 days without eating at least some of what I like...or constantly counting calories and nutrients. To me, that sounds like torture—a life full of math without my favorite foods.

However, the science behind the plan is really very convincing...but very hard to test on people (at least outside of a strictly controlled environment). This diet has 30% to 40% fewer calories than a normal diet, with all of the necessary nutrients to sustain life included. It appears to lengthen the life of practically every animal it has been tested on, from fruit flies to mice. The testing has now progressed to primates—and while this type of diet does seem to slow at least some aging processes, the results aren't yet conclusive.

While I wholeheartedly recommend a healthy diet—with lots of fruits, vegetables, whole grains, lean proteins, and healty fats—I can't really wrap my mind around what sounds like starvation rations. Even if the plan really will work for people, I don't know many (if any) people who could really stick with it for the long haul.

The Dental-Health Connection

A healthy-*looking* smile is easier to get than ever. We have braces, crowns, whiteners, brighteners...everything you need to make sure your teeth look great. Oral health is another thing entirely, and now we know about its very close links to aging and systemic disease. The latest studies tell us that dental health is directly connected to overall health and that poor dental health can cause serious whole-body problems. Some of the conditions associated with poor dental health include:

- diabetes
- heart attack
- stroke
- chronic inflammation
- bacterial infections
- respiratory infections

The Fluoride Myth

How did an industrial poison become a key player in dental health? Marketing. Most people in the United States—including most dental professionals—believe that fluoride is crucial for stronger, healthier teeth. In fact, the opposite may be true. New studies indicate that fluroide may destroy your dental health, and even weaken your bones. Additional evidence shows that people who get too much fluoride get white splotches on their teeth, giving their smiles a mottled appearance that can't be corrected with normal teeth-whitening methods.

It all starts with gum disease. The mildest, "just-starting-out" version is called gingivitis, and that shows up as swollen red (sometimes bleeding) gums. Left untreated, the condition deteriorates until you face chronic inflammation, frequent infections, and even bone loss. Here's how: Bacteria along the gum line break down tissue, allowing even more bacteria to get in, which breaks down the tissue even further—it's a self-perpetuating cycle. Next, the invading bacteria cross into your bloodstream, where it can cause whole-body diseases and activate a strong immune response. That can lead to even more inflammation, which may accelerate the aging process.

There are simple solutions to this problem: Take better care of your teeth and gums. Brush and floss regularly. Get to the dentist at least twice a year. Gargle a couple of times a week with straight hydrogen peroxide (making sure not to swallow any). And stock up on the nutrients that contribute to good dental health, like calcium and folic acid.

Longevity Genes

Since decoding the human genome, scientists have been making DNA-related discoveries left and right. One of the more exciting research areas involve a small band of genes that controls our bodies' defense mechanisms and may radically extend life and promote good health. Once the secrets of these genes are unraveled, we just may have the means to live longer and healthier lives.

Specific genes get their own names, which usually sound like secret passwords and sometimes like biblical or mythological beings. Longevity genes—or at least the ones researchers believe have ties to long-life expectancies—come with such diverse names as SIRT1, Methusaleh, and Klotho, and Clock. Some of these genes suppress activities that cause age-related changes. Others keep youth-promoting processes running longer.

The Longevity-Gene Pool

Though actual therapies are a long way off, here are some of the specific genes being explored by researchers right now:

- SIRT1 has been shown to extend life by 30% in yeast, worms, and flies by influencing stress responses and metabolism.
- Methusaleh added 35% more time to a fly's life when researchers suppressed the gene's activity.

- Klotho let mice live up to 31% longer through its regulation of insulin, IGF-1 (the insulin-like growth factor), and vitamin D. Messing with this gene could cause insulin resistance, which could lead to blood-sugar problems.
- Clock genes influence the production of coenzyme Q10. Reducing their activity added 30% more time to the lifespan of worms.

Flipping Switches

Most of today's antiaging research revolves around specific genes, and what happens when scientists turn these genes on and off. And in most cases, the scientists have no idea what the repercussions might be when those switches get flipped. Altering a single gene could have monumental effects on your life and health, far beyond the intent of the treatment.

On top of that, genes are only a piece of the longevity puzzle. Lifestyle choices may be equally—or even more—important. Regardless of a person's genetic makeup, things like smoking, poor diet, low activity level, and constant stress can shorten his lifespan. That makes a 100% focus on genetics unwise at best.

Lengthening Telomeres

Telomeres are little cap-like sections at the ends of our chromosomes, sort of like the plastic ends on your shoelaces that are there to keep them from fraying. Every single time a cell divides, its telomeres get a little shorter—until they eventually disappear and the cell dies off. Short telomeres are linked to aging. And some scientists believe that lengthening those little DNA strands can lengthen life as well.

So far, we know about one thing that seems to counteract this shortening process—an enzyme called telomerase. When cells are young, telomerase prevents the telomeres from too much wearing away. As the cells keep dividing, though, the telomerase depletes and the telomeres shorten.

In the lab, researchers have been able to keep telomeres intact and maintain cell division much longer than normal by adding some extra telomerase into the mix. But excess telomerase has a dark side—it's also connected to cancer, as cancer cells turn on this enzyme to keep themselves from dying. So far, though, the addition of telomerase to healthy cells hasn't brought on cancer...at least not in the lab...but we still don't know what will happen to people when this substance is added to the mix.

Your Next Step

Antiaging research continues in virtually all directions, from gene therapies to hormone replenishment to near-starvation diets. As the research continues, I continue to give advice that I know works to help people live longer, healthier lives—the recommendations you've read throughout this book.

Start now! Take the steps to reset your biological clock right now. You'll feel better, stronger...less pain, more energy...more youthful than you have in years. No matter how old you are now, you can start reversing the symptoms of aging and erasing the signs. All you have to do is take that first step, backward to a more vital you.

Next Stop, Immortality?

Back in the 1600s, the average Joe lived about 30 years. By the late 1990s, the average lifespan had more than doubled to about 76 years. Some scientists believe that average will move up again by the end of this century, at a much more rapid pace. A hopeful handful think that by eliminating all of the normal aging processes and finding ways to repair cell damage, people could live for 1,000 years. And others believe that average human lifespan will top out at 90 years. Who's right? Only time will tell.

INDEX

C

D

E